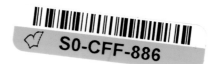
THE OFFICIAL UNIVERSAL WORKOUT BOOK

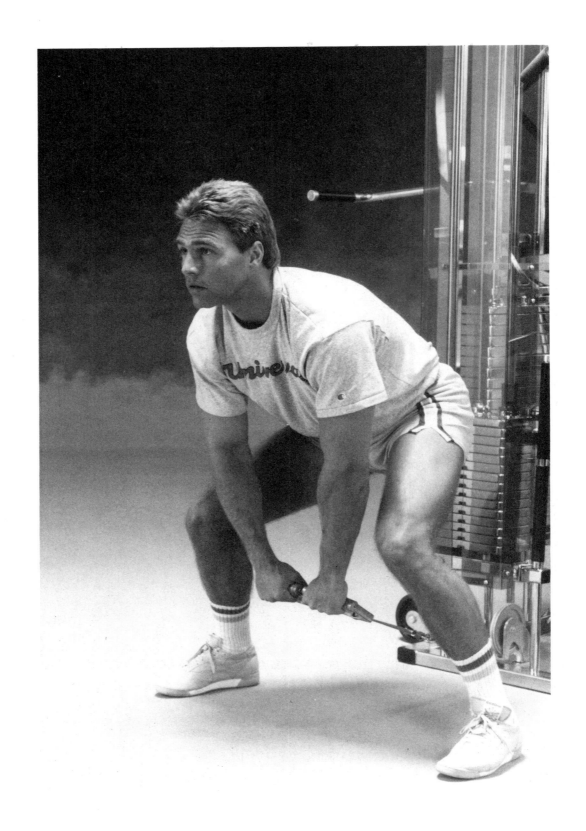

THE OFFICIAL UNIVERSAL WORKOUT BOOK

BY CHUCK COKER AND FRANK SMITH
WITH JIM NELSON
PHOTOGRAPHS BY ROD BRADLEY

A PERIGEE/MOUNTAIN LION BOOK

Perigee Books
are published by
The Putnam Publishing Group
200 Madison Avenue
New York, NY 10016

Library of Congress Cataloging-in-Publication Data

Coker, Chuck.
    The official Universal workout book.

    "A Perigee/Mountain Lion book."
    1. Universal weight training equipment.   2. Weight
training.   I. Smith, Frank, date.   II. Nelson, Jim,
date.   III. Universal Gym Equipment, Inc.
IV. Title.
GV548.U54C64   1988   796.4′1′028   87-30364
ISBN 0-399-51399-X

Printed in the United States of America
1 2 3 4 5 5 6 7 8 10

Contents

	Introduction	7
1	Fitness Is Universal	9
2	What Is Total Body Fitness?	13
3	Universal Training Principles and Fundamentals	27
4	Varying the Workout	33
5	Warming Up	37
6	Training and Building the Legs and Hips	49
7	Training and Building the Upper Torso, Arms, and Neck	67
8	Training and Building the Abdominals and Lower Back	135
9	Hand Strength	163
10	Workout Routines and Circuit Training	175
11	Aerobics and Universal Workouts	181
12	What's Ahead in Universal Fitness	185
	Appendix Universal Workout Record	189

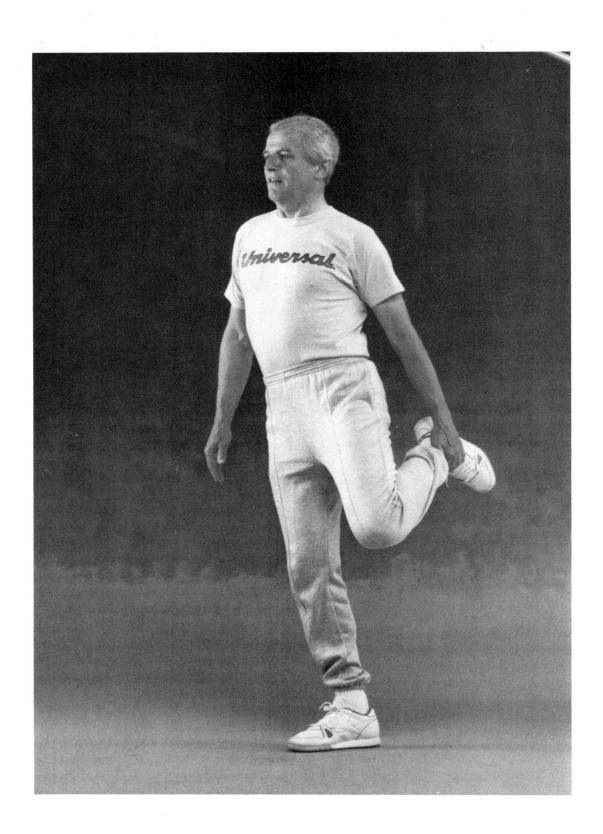

INTRODUCTION

This book is for you, whether you're young or old, male or female; whether you're athletically inclined or a beginning enthusiast; whether you're in good shape or in no particular shape at all. It's for anyone who's looking for a complete exercise program that has been time-tested through years of experience.

Universal has been in existence since 1957. Today millions of people train with Universal equipment in more than 120 countries around the globe. Universal equipment is popular because it *works.* And Universal's continued research in biomechanics and exercise physiology ensures that it will remain at the forefront of the fitness movement.

The Official Universal Workout Book is a primer on weight training using Universal equipment. The book will show you how to tailor Universal exercise programs to meet your individual fitness goals and your lifestyle.

One note of caution, however: Before you begin this or any other exercise program, you should get a complete physical examination from your doctor, especially if you're over thirty years old or have a chronic medical condition, such as diabetes, high blood pressure, or heart disease. Be sure to read the manufacturer's instructions before using any equipment.

The Official Universal Workout Book will help you get started on the road to a healthier, more vital you. We welcome your comments and suggestions as you progress with the workout programs.

Chuck Coker
Frank Smith

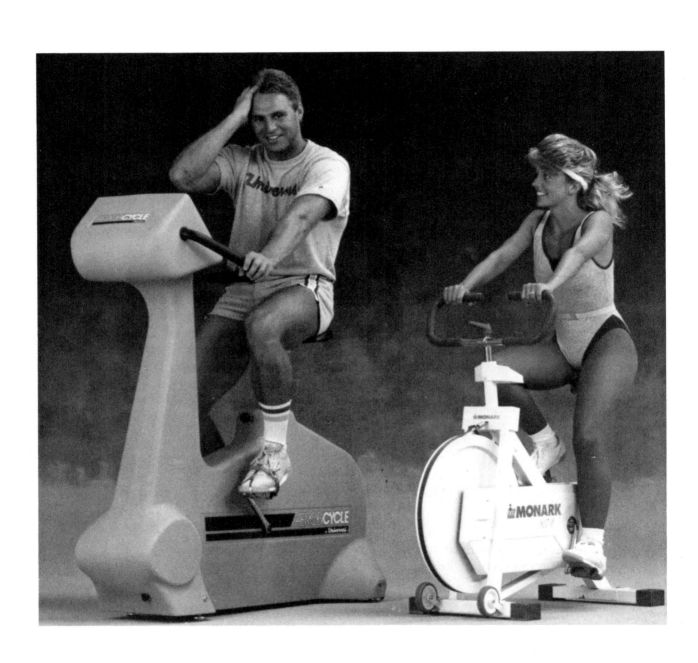

1

Fitness Is Universal

Harold Zinkin and Milt McAleece started the Universal Athletic Sales Company more than twenty-five years ago. Harold Zinkin, the first Mr. California, had owned and operated numerous health clubs in the late forties and fifties. He and Milt McAleece were later joined by Chuck Coker, a one-time United States decathlon team member, and a successful college coach who had instituted weight training classes in 1951 in the California schools. All three recognized the need for a new system of physical conditioning to replace barbells and dumbbells in schools and health clubs across the country, with which people working out sometimes injured themselves by dropping the weights accidentally because of muscular fatigue. They developed a revolutionary, fixed-weight, four-station weight training machine that combined bench press, leg press, high/low pulley and shoulder press functions. This was the first Universal machine.

Persuading people to use their revolutionary invention was not easy at first, despite the obvious safety and workout advantages. But the founders were determined. In one year, Chuck Coker drove 120,000 miles with one of the prototype machines, demonstrating the benefits of the Universal machine at schools, clubs, hospitals, police departments—wherever people were interested. Slowly but surely skeptics became converts, and Universal's exercise equipment took the athletic and health communities by storm.

The key to Universal's success has been its continued dedication to research. Early on, Universal recognized that equipment should be built to meet its users' specifications, rather than forcing its users to fit the machine's specifications. Universal was the first company in its field to employ computer-bio-mechanical research in the development of functional exercise equipment. Universal's new generation of dynamic variable resistance (DVR) machines evolved out of this research.

The DVR Difference

Unlike barbells, Universal's DVR machines automatically and progressively adjust the weight resistance a person works against to accommodate the body's changing leverage during each lifting stroke. Although barbells require near maximal effort from the starting point of an exercise through midrange of the lifting motion, from there to lockout, the end of the motion, the muscles are exerting much less effort—they are coasting. DVR machines use either a DVR lifting arm or a specially developed DVR *cam* to help the person using the machine maintain the same relative degree of muscular exertion through the full range of motion. This makes your workout more effective and efficient.

THE SCIENCE OF CIRCUIT TRAINING

Originally pioneered at the University of Leeds, England, circuit training was first adapted by Universal to provide conditioning for high-strength development, balanced conditioning, and aerobic weight training. Universal was one of the few companies to sponsor additional research on the benefits of circuit training, which it continues today.

The Universal system utilizes a series of resistive exercise stations, which, when used in a predetermined sequence called a *circuit,* exercise all the body's major muscle groups. Circuit training offers a host of advantages:

- Balanced conditioning—Muscle groups work in pairs. Universal's single-station and multistation machine circuits provide exercises for the muscle groups that work antagonistically to one another, as many muscles on the front and back of the body do.
- Efficient use of time—Universal's selectorized equipment makes it quick and easy to change weights on each station. In addition, Universal's design makes spotters unnecessary, allowing a large group of people to get a complete workout in a short amount of time.

- Individualized progress—You can assess your own development and adjust the intensity of the circuit accordingly.
- Increased motivation—The movement from one station to another introduces an element of variety that is missing from a sequence of exercises performed in one location.

Let's take a quick look at each of Universal's conditioning circuits.

ANTAGONISTIC MUSCLE CIRCUIT—FOR STRENGTH DEVELOPMENT

The Universal Antagonistic Muscle Circuit alternately exercises muscle groups that work (contract) in direct opposition to each other (antagonist-agonist).

For example, a biceps exercise would be immediately followed with a triceps exercise. Heavy resistance and a low number of repetitions (for example, 70–80 percent of maximum lift with five to seven reps) are used throughout the circuit, with almost no pause between stations. This approach enhances your muscle strength gains greatly.

PERIPHERAL HEART ACTION CIRCUIT—FOR BALANCED CONDITIONING

The Universal Peripheral Heart Action Circuit alternates upper- and lower-body exercises throughout the entire circuit, with moderate resistance and a high number of repetitions (for example, 40–60 percent of maximum lift with twelve to fifteen reps).

AEROBIC SUPER CIRCUIT—FOR HIGH-INTENSITY AEROBIC WEIGHT TRAINING

The Universal Aerobic Super Circuit combines the exercises in the Peripheral Heart Action Circuit with thirty seconds of aerobic activity (such as using a stationary cycle or jumping rope) between stations. The resistance and repetitions should be the same as for the peripheral heart circuit. The result: total body fitness.

WHY YOU NEED MORE THAN AEROBICS

Thousands of Americans are avid walkers, joggers, and bicyclists, enjoying the benefits of cardiovascular exercise. But aerobics are not enough to develop good overall conditioning. Aerobics do a good job of conditioning the heart and lungs, but they fall short of providing total body fitness. They fail to develop the upper body sufficiently and they leave some of the muscles in the legs under-developed. For example, bicycling over-develops the calf and quadriceps muscles but short-changes the hamstrings. This imbalance can lead to injury in other activities.

We're not saying you should abandon your aerobics program if you are a jogger or cyclist, but you should supplement it with an overall conditioning program like those described in the *Official Universal Workout Book.* Beginners, especially, should begin a resistive exercise program before they start jogging. Strong muscles can withstand the jarring impact of running. Weak muscles cannot. Instead of playing yourself into shape, as happens too often in American sports, you should get into shape to play. Integrating Universal's programs with aerobic training is a dramatic combination that will give you the kind of body you want—inside and out.

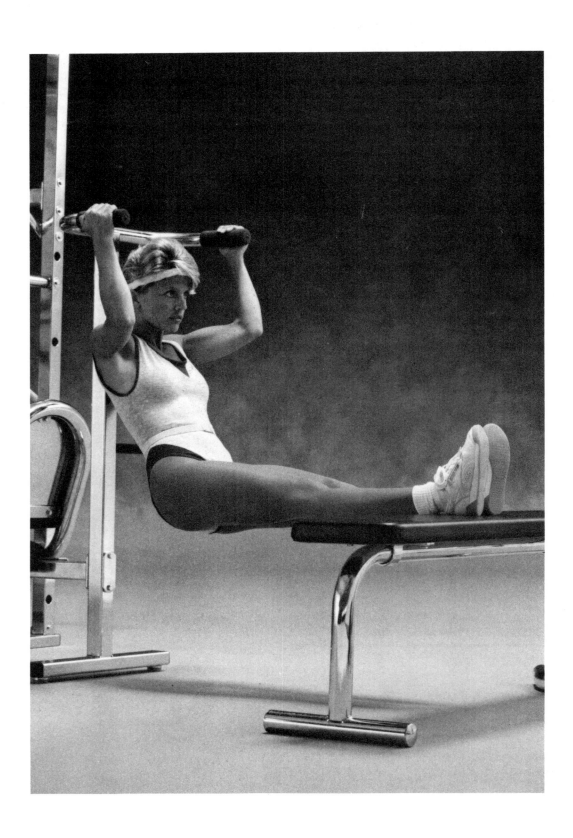

2

WHAT IS TOTAL BODY FITNESS?

MYTHS AND MISCONCEPTIONS

The exercise field is rife with misinformation. Part of Universal's mission is to separate fact from fallacy through research. In that vein, let's expose some all-too-common fitness myths.

AEROBICS IS THE ONLY FITNESS PROGRAM YOU NEED

Granted, if your heart isn't in good shape it doesn't really matter what the rest of your body looks like. But you still need more than aerobics for a full and active life. Sports, for example, usually require a good measure of strength and flexibility as well. Weight training is especially important to help prevent sports injuries. And most people want the kind of musculature that only an all-around conditioning program can provide.

IF YOU'RE OVER FORTY, YOU'RE OVER THE HILL

A scientifically designed exercise program can help you turn back the clock. Although your chronological age may be forty-three, you may have the body of a thirty-year-old. Most of the decline in strength and aerobic capacity seen in older people comes from disuse of the body rather than as a natural part of the aging process. Bodies were made to be used. A sedentary lifestyle is one of the most insidious and harmful forms of abuse that you can subject your body to.

EXERCISE IS FOR ATHLETES ONLY

Exercise is for everyone, men, women, young, old, those who are in shape and those who are not. Universal's programs allow you to work at your own pace toward your own individual fitness goals.

BIG MUSCLES MEAN YOU'RE PHYSICALLY FIT

Big muscles mean you have big muscles. If you choose form over function, you're neglecting your body. A fitness program should also improve strength, muscle endurance, flexibility, aerobic fitness, and body composition.

MAJOR COMPONENTS OF FITNESS

Total body fitness is more than just how efficiently our body parts function — how much we can lift, how far we can run, how far we can bend. Total body fitness means having the strength and energy to do the things that are important to you at work, at home, and at play. But to get the most out of life, you have to be willing to invest the time to give yourself the body you deserve.

Total body fitness involves five areas:

- Cardiorespiratory endurance or aerobic fitness.
- Strength, tone, muscle balance, and endurance.
- Flexibility.
- Muscle mass/body fat ratio.
- Muscular balance.

Let's look at each of them.

AEROBIC FITNESS

If you are aerobically fit, your lungs and circulatory system work together to efficiently circulate blood and oxygen throughout the body. The major parts of the circulatory system are the heart, arteries, veins, and capillaries. The circulatory system's job is to supply blood to all tissues in the body, providing us with the nutrients and oxygen necessary for the production of energy. Simultaneously, the circulatory system removes the waste products.

Your key to aerobic fitness is an efficient heart. The heart is a muscle. As with all muscles, exercise improves the heart's ability to do work. But in order to strengthen your heart, the exercise has to be *aerobic* exercise like running, swimming, or Universal's Aerobic Super Circuit Program. These activities must be performed for at least twenty minutes and must elevate the heart rate to the individual's training range. These activities are rhythmic in nature and use the large muscles in the body; most important, they condition the heart to function efficiently. How? Aerobic exercise causes the heart's muscle contractions to become more powerful, forcing it to empty itself more completely at each stroke, increasing both the stroke volume and the cardiac output. This increase in strength and efficiency enables the heart to circulate more blood while beating less frequently. That's why runners often have heart rates ten to twenty beats per minute slower than the general population. A strong, efficient heart can deliver a larger blood flow to the muscles, ensuring an adequate supply of fuel and oxygen, which permits you to perform better.

Copious Capillaries. If veins and arteries are the interstate highways of the circulatory system, capillaries are the back roads. Veins and arteries transport blood most of the way through the body, but capillaries are responsible for bringing the vital oxygen and nutrients to their final destination — the muscles and organs. Aerobic exercise can increase the number of capillaries within a muscle by up to 50 percent, allowing more blood to get where it's needed. In addition, a larger network of tiny blood vessels can sometimes prevent damage to the body when an artery gets blocked by providing a detour around the blockage.

Better Blood Cells. Regular aerobic exercise can double the number of red corpuscles in the blood. This change in blood composition is significant because corpuscles carry hemoglobin, which unites with oxygen, bringing that vital element to the muscles and organs. Higher levels of hemoglobin can vastly improve your endurance and increase your mental and physical alertness.

Livelier Lungs. The heart and our blood cells aren't the only things that benefit from regular aerobic exercise. The respiratory system does too. Generally, it takes six to eight weeks of aerobic training to bring your respiratory system near maximum efficiency. As lung capacity and muscular efficiency increases, the heartrate and respiratory rate during exercise decreases. This will decrease your oxygen consumption and carbon dioxide production. Heavy training can reduce the amount of air you need to take in per minute by as much as 25 percent for a given load.

THE MUSCLE TRIO: STRENGTH, TONE, AND ENDURANCE

Strength is a measure of your body's ability to lift, push, or pull. Strength can be improved through either static (isometric) or dynamic (isotonic) exercises. Static exercises, as their name implies, involve muscle contractions that are not accompanied by movement. Static contractions of five to ten seconds *will* strengthen muscle, but the gains are probably restricted to that particular joint angle. On the other hand, dynamic exercises, which are accompanied by movement, strengthen the muscle through the full range of motion. For this reason, Universal programs rely on this type of exercise.

For total body fitness, the muscles in your body should be strong enough for you to do the things you want to do, whether that means hitting a baseball or lifting the spare tire out of your trunk.

Tone is the glamour part of muscular fitness. It's what gives muscles their definition. Bodies without muscle tone sag and lack definition. In short, muscle tone is a measure of the firmness of muscle

tissue. (Note: proper posture will help develop muscle tone.)

Why is muscle tone so important? Because appearances matter so much in our culture. A strong, well-toned body exudes confidence and ability, which is an asset in all aspects of our lives, both work and play. All of Universal's exercise programs help develop and maintain good muscle tone.

Muscle endurance may not be as glamorous as muscle tone, but it's a lot more useful. Muscle endurance is a measure of your muscles' ability to perform work over a period of time. Running, swimming, and chopping wood are all activities that rely on good muscle endurance. Moms and dads need muscle endurance to run after their kids (who seem to be blessed with an inordinate supply of endurance). Tennis players need muscle endurance to play their best in a long match. Football players need muscle endurance to compete in the final quarter. Anyone who wants to maintain an active lifestyle needs good muscle endurance.

FLEXIBILITY

Flexibility is the ability of muscles and tendons to move through a normal range of motion around a joint. Being flexible is essential for total fitness and total success of your exercise program because flexible muscles are less prone to injury and give you a greater range of motion. To increase your flexibility, you should stretch the muscles that cross the joints and attach to the bones. When muscles have been systematically stretched, they can contract over a longer period of time.

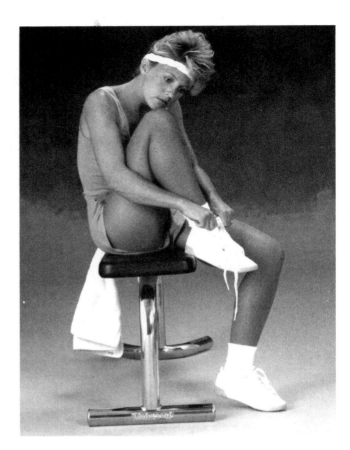

MUSCLE MASS VERSUS BODY FAT

Besides bones, our bodies are composed mainly of muscle and fat. Muscle is biologically active and performs a function in the body. Fat just weighs you down. For that reason, most researchers and physicians feel that the percentage of body fat is a better indicator of health than is total body weight. Obesity places a strain on the heart and is linked with diabetes, high blood pressure, and heart disease.

Everyone needs some fat. Without it, there would be nothing to cushion the body's delicate organs. Men, for example, require at least 4 percent fat. Women, on the other hand, need at least 9 percent. The average for young active adults ranges from 15 percent for men to 22 percent for women. The average for active, older adults ranges from 18 to 24 percent. Goals for *optimal* fitness would be 10 percent body fat for men and 18 percent for women. In the next section, you'll learn how to determine your percentage of body fat.

ASSESSING YOUR FITNESS LEVEL

Before you can design your fitness program, you must know where you stand now. The first stop should be your doctor's office for a complete physical. Professor P. O. Ostrand, noted Swedish exercise physiologist, says, "Anyone who is in doubt about the condition of his health should consult his physician, but as a general rule, moderate activity is less harmful to the health than inactivity." You could also put it this way: A medical exam is more urgent for those who plan to remain inactive than for those who intend to get into good physical shape. Even so, if you're over thirty-five years old, you should consider arranging for a stress test at a sports medicine clinic. There, doctors will monitor your heart and oxygen consumption as you walk on a treadmill, looking for any hidden abnormalities. If you pass, you'll feel that much more confident as you start your exercise program. If the stress test turns up something, you'll want to know so you can tailor your exercise program accordingly.

You can get a good idea of your fitness level by doing the tests outlined in the following sections. The tests will tell you how your fitness level relates to that of the general population, and they will provide you with reference points so you can gauge the improvement in your fitness levels.

BENCH STEP TEST

F. Kasch and J. Boyer have developed a three-minute step test that measures cardiovascular fitness. It requires considerable exertion. If you experience chest pains or serious shortness of breath, stop the test immediately. The test requires the following equipment:

- A twelve-inch bench for stepping.
- A clock with sweep second hand or stopwatch for timing the test and counting your heart rate.
- A metronome to help you maintain cadence and proper stepping rate.
- A stethoscope to count your heart rate during the recovery period. (The stethoscope provides the most accurate measure of your heart rate, but you can also take your pulse on your wrist.)

The purpose of the step test is to measure the heart rate in the recovery period following three minutes of stepping; the results can be used to estimate maximum oxygen intake.

To perform the step test, step on the bench with both feet, right foot first.

Then step off the bench, right foot first. Repeat the action until the time is up. The rate of stepping is twenty-four steps per minute. Immediately after the three minutes of stepping, sit down. After five seconds, count your heart rate for sixty seconds by placing the stethoscope over your heart and counting the beats. The chart below shows how to evaluate your performance.

THREE-MINUTE STEP TEST

Males		Females
Heart Rate		Heart Rate
71 or less	Excellent	96 or less
72–102	Good	97–127
103–117	Average	128–142
118–147	Fair	143–171
148 or more	Poor	172 or more

SIT-UP TEST FOR DYNAMIC STRENGTH

How strong are your abdominal muscles? How much endurance do they have? This test will show you.

Lie on your back, knees bent, feet flat on the floor, and hands interlocked behind the neck. Have someone hold your feet down. Try to do as many correct sit-ups as possible in one minute. Your elbows should touch your knees on the up phase and your back should touch the floor before you start the next sit-up. Don't pull on your head or jerk when sitting up; this can strain the muscles in your neck and back. Remember to breathe throughout the test. The following chart shows typical performance levels for healthy adults. If scored in the 90 percentile range, that means your performance was better than 90 percent of those tested.

MUSCULAR ENDURANCE
ONE-MINUTE SIT-UP—NUMBER

FEMALE

AGE

%	<20	20–29	30–39	40–49	50–59	60+		
99	>54.8	>51.0	>42.0	>37.5	>30.1	>28.0		Superior
95	54.8	51.0	42.0	37.5	30.1	28.0		
90	54.8	48.5	40.4	34.0	29.0	26.0		
85	48.8	45.3	37.5	32.0	26.3	19.9		Excellent
80	45.6	44.0	35.0	29.0	24.0	17.2		
75	40.0	42.0	33.0	28.0	22.0	14.5		
70	37.6	41.0	32.0	27.0	22.0	12.0		Good
65	37.0	39.3	30.0	25.0	21.0	12.0		
60	36.2	38.0	29.0	24.0	20.0	11.2		
55	34.8	37.0	28.0	23.0	18.9	9.7		
50	34.0	34.5	27.0	22.0	17.0	8.0		Fair
45	34.0	34.0	26.0	21.0	16.0	8.0		
40	31.6	32.0	25.0	20.0	14.0	5.8		
35	29.6	31.0	24.0	19.0	12.0	4.5		
30	29.0	29.5	22.0	17.0	12.0	4.0		Poor
25	29.0	28.0	21.0	15.5	11.0	3.8		
20	28.2	27.0	20.0	14.0	10.0	3.0		
15	26.8	24.0	18.0	12.5	7.0	2.1		
10	25.2	22.5	15.0	10.0	5.8	1.0		Very Poor
5	25.2	18.3	11.0	6.5	5.0	.6		
1	<25.2	<18.3	<11.0	<6.5	<5.0	<.6		
							Total	
Number Tested	15	144	289	249	137	26	860	

Information courtesy of the Institute for Aerobics Research

MUSCULAR ENDURANCE
ONE-MINUTE SIT-UP — NUMBER

MALE

AGE

%	<20	20–29	30–39	40–49	50–59	60+		
99	>61.7	>55.0	>51.0	>47.0	>43.0	>39.0		Superior
95	61.7	55.0	51.0	47.0	43.0	39.0		
90	55.0	51.7	48.0	43.0	39.0	35.0		
85	53.0	49.0	45.0	40.0	36.0	31.0		Excellent
80	50.6	47.0	43.0	39.0	35.0	30.0		
75	50.0	45.8	42.0	37.0	33.0	28.0		
70	48.0	45.0	41.0	36.0	31.0	26.0		Good
65	47.6	44.0	40.0	35.0	30.0	24.0		
60	47.0	42.0	39.0	34.0	28.0	22.0		
55	46.0	41.0	37.0	32.0	27.0	21.3		
50	44.5	40.0	36.0	31.0	26.0	20.0		Fair
45	42.0	39.0	35.0	30.0	25.0	19.0		
40	41.0	38.0	35.0	29.0	24.0	19.0		
35	39.4	37.0	33.0	28.0	22.0	18.0		
30	38.0	35.0	32.0	27.0	21.0	17.0		Poor
25	37.0	35.0	31.0	26.0	20.0	16.0		
20	36.0	33.0	30.0	24.0	19.0	15.0		
15	34.1	32.0	28.0	22.0	17.0	13.0		
10	33.1	30.0	26.0	20.0	15.0	10.0		Very Poor
5	26.8	27.0	23.0	17.0	12.0	7.0		
1	<26.8	<27.0	<23.0	<17.0	<12.0	<7.0		
							Total	
Number Tested	46	312	1,431	1,558	919	205	4,471	

Information courtesy of the Institute for Aerobics Research

PUSH-UPS

Push-ups provide a quick assessment of upper-body strength. Do as many push-ups as you can in one minute without stopping. With your body parallel to the floor and your arms extended, lower your chest to the floor. Make sure you keep your back straight, and your head up as you do them. Your chest should touch the floor every time. Women can perform the push-ups with their knees touching the ground. Score yourself as follows:

	Males	*Females*
High	50 or more	30 or more
Average	20–49	10–29
Low	0–19	0–9

FLEXIBILITY TEST

Flexibility is included in total fitness assessment because of widespread problems of low-back pain and joint soreness. Many of these problems are related to sedentary living. Flexibility is defined as the range of possible movement in a joint or group of joints.

No general flexibility test measures the flexibility of all joints; however, the trunk flexion, or the sit and reach test, serves as an important measure of hip and back flexibility.

Sit on the floor, legs straight, feet together. Bend forward and reach as far as you can past your toes. Don't bounce during the exercise. Have a partner measure the distance you can reach past your toes. Score yourself as follows:

Excellent	8 inches or more past your toes
Good	2–8 inches past your toes
Average	Touch toes
Poor	Unable to touch your toes.

BODY FAT MEASUREMENT

For a rough indication of whether you're overweight, try pinching your fat (don't pinch the muscle) on the area around your triceps. If you can hold more than an inch between your thumb and index finger, you should think about going on a diet and exercise plan. But remember, this test is only a rough indication of your fat level. Calipers provide a more precise indication of fat levels, providing the person doing the reading has been trained to use them properly.

VITAL STATISTICS

Pulse Rate. Your resting pulse rate is a good indicator of your cardiovascular fitness. You can take your pulse in any one of three ways: Place your hand over your heart and count the number of beats; place your finger on your windpipe at the neck and move it to the groove on either side; or place your middle finger on the inside of your wrist at the base of your thumb and move it about an inch up your forearm. Count the beats for ten seconds and then multiply that number by six, which gives you a heart rate for one minute. That is your Resting Heart Rate, and it will become a point of reference in measuring your improvement in aerobic capacity as you continue training.

As that capacity improves, the Resting Heart Rate will diminish, because the heart will become more efficient and stronger in its capacity to pump blood throughout your system (see Appendix for further details).

Blood Pressure. Have your doctor take your blood pressure. Anything above 140/90 is considered high. But did you know that a sensible exercise program, especially one that emphasizes aerobics, can help you lower your blood pressure? Ask your doctor. It's true.

Girth Measurements. It's time to get out the tape measure and record your chest, waist, and hip measurements. If you're especially concerned about another body part, such as the thighs or biceps, record that too. These measurements are important because the weight scale is not a reliable way to judge if you're losing fat. A higher reading may just mean that you're adding muscle, which is denser than fat. The tape measure (and your mirror) will reveal the true story.

Weight. Record your weight, but don't be obsessed by the scale. Remember its limitations as a judge of your fat levels.

DEVELOPING YOUR PRESCRIPTION FOR FITNESS

You know best the kind of fitness program you need. The first thing you should do is take a long hard look at yourself in the mirror. Do you like what you see? Are there areas that need to be firmed up or trimmed down?

Now think about your lifestyle. Do you get winded going up a couple of flights of stairs? If so, your aerobic capacity probably needs some work. Do your muscles lack definition? You'll want to work at toning your muscles. Do you suffer from chronic fatigue? The remedy isn't to get more sack time. No, you'll want a program that emphasizes cardiorespiratory fitness and muscular endurance. Think about where you need improvement as you read through the following sections, which discuss the elements that make up a fitness program.

COMBINE AEROBIC AND WEIGHT TRAINING

Everyone needs a solid base of aerobic exercise. The question is whether you want to get it through Universal's Super Circuit Program or by combining an aer-

obic activity with your Universal workout. If you enjoy jogging, swimming, or bicycling, it makes sense to work these activities into your workout schedule. You'll benefit from the variety of exercising outside the gym, and it's likely that your weight-training program will help prevent injuries in your chosen activity. Aerobic activities are best at exercising the heart, but as all-over muscle conditioners, generally they're not as good. Typically, they overcondition certain muscle groups and undercondition others.

EXERCISE AND CONTROLLING WEIGHT/FAT METABOLISM

Diets alone don't work. If they did, there wouldn't be such a profusion of diet books, each one claiming to be the final answer for getting weight off and keeping it off. Diets don't work because your body reacts to reduced food intake by slowing its metabolism. Therefore, you can eat less and still not lose weight.

The answer to slimming down is to combine a sensible diet with an exercise program. Exercise not only burns calories while you're performing the activity, it also keeps burning calories for several hours afterward. Exercise also keeps your metabolism running high if you cut down your food intake.

Unlike diets, exercise builds muscles to help your body look as good as it can. Exercise is the key to getting—and keeping—the look you want.

SET YOUR GOALS AND DEVELOP STRATEGIES

Your workout program can be boring drudgery or a wonderful revitalizer that prepares you for the rest of your day (or night). It all depends on your attitude. In your spare moments, picture yourself as the Adonis or Aphrodite that you deserve to be. Call that picture up when-

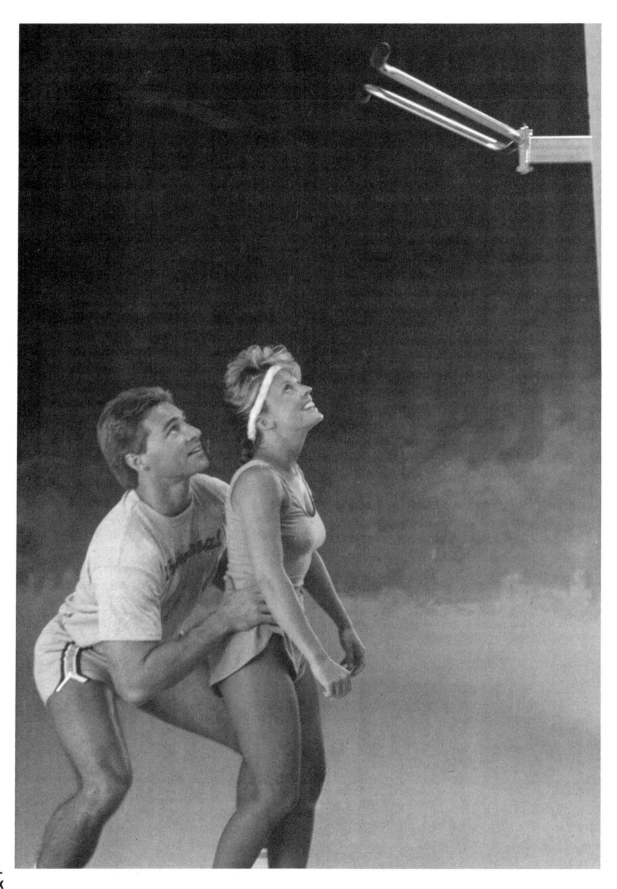

ever you feel tempted to skip your workout. We guarantee that if you remain faithful to your exercise program, you can achieve the goal you've set for yourself, whether it's to lose weight, increase muscle mass, firm up, increase strength, or improve your figure. The key to a successful fitness program is 90 percent mental and 10 percent physical. So project a positive mental image of what you want to be and dedicate yourself to that goal.

Don't compromise your attitude during your workout. Instead of counting the repetitions in each set and thinking "thank goodness that's over" when you're finished, concentrate on the muscle groups you're using. Concentrate on including as many muscle fibers as possible, even when the resistance is light. Mentally concentrate on those muscle groups with as much intensity as you can muster. You'll be surprised. This increased mental focus can improve your results by 25 percent or more.

Throughout your workout, remind yourself how pumped up you will feel once you've completed it, ready to tackle anything. That good feeling that your workout gives you has a physical basis. Intense physical activity causes endorphins, a natural "feel-good" hormone, to be released in the brain.

REMIND YOURSELF OF THE BENEFITS

As you progress with your training program, you will see improvements in many areas: cardiovascular endurance, strength, muscle stamina, flexibility, and self-confidence. In addition, an improved circulation system delivers more oxygen and glucose to the brain, making you more alert and better able to cope with the stresses and challenges of life. But to get these benefits, you must stay committed to your workouts. If you cheat, your body will reflect that. But if you remain dedicated to fitness, your

finely toned body will display that fact proudly. The sky is the limit, the rest is up to you.

BE REALISTIC

The hard-work part scares many people off the exercise routine. Start slowly! In the first six to eight weeks, your body must adapt to your new workout regimen. Listen to your body, and don't push yourself beyond what's reasonable. The key to a successful workout program is to keep at it, not pushing yourself so hard that you get injured.

THE POWER OF PARTNERS

Finding a partner who is as committed as you are to your workout program can help you stay motivated. Occasionally, everyone is tempted to skip a workout. A rough day at work, pouring rain that you don't want to battle to get to the gym, or just a serious case of the blahs can all make you say "Why bother?" A partner can keep you psyched up and your program on track. "C'mon," your partner will tell you, "once you get to the gym, you'll be glad you did." And you will.

If your partner is always canceling on you, it's time to get a new partner. Try to find someone whose enthusiasm level, goals, and body type match yours. It's easy to get discouraged when your partner is able to lift grand pianos and you're still struggling with the piano bench. But when your abilities are on a par with your partner's, you'll spur each other on to greater and greater achievements.

RECORDING WORKOUT DATA

In the Appendix, we've provided a blank workout form. Make one copy of the form and write the exercises in your program along the left side. Use this form as your original. Make a few copies to keep handy for recording your workout data.

As you fill up each form, file it for reference later. When you see how much you've improved, you'll be that much more motivated to continue with your program. If you don't see the kind of improvement you'd like in some areas, you may want to readjust your program by changing the weight, the number of reps, or the number of sets in those particular exercises.

NUTRITIONAL GUIDELINES

Heart disease, diabetes, and cancer have all been linked to the foods we eat. If your diet consists primarily of high-fat foods like french fries and refined carbohydrates like ice cream and soft drinks, you must develop the will power to control your eating habits. Build up your arms and push away from the table.

The real reason for eating is to build up our body chemistry. Do you eat for that purpose? For example, do you eat a hot-fudge sundae because it will build up your body chemistry? No, you eat it because you like it. The brain needs to be reprogrammed for good nutrition.

Most information on nutrition is provided by companies that want us to buy their products. But the sad fact is that most of the food we eat has little nutritional value.

THE MAKINGS OF A GOOD DIET

For proper nutrition, we need adequate amounts of protein, carbohydrates, fats, vitamins, minerals, and fiber. The word "protein" comes from the Greek and means "of first importance." It's an aptly named substance. Our muscles, skin, hair, heart, lungs, brain, and nerves are all made of protein. Hormones, the chemical regulators of body processes,

and enzymes, the spark plugs of chemical reactions, are also protein.

Every cell in the body is replaced every 160 days. The cells of the vital organs turn over much faster. The cells of the liver, for example, are replaced in its entirety in about two weeks. The heart, muscles, kidneys, glands, the walls of the stomach, and the veins and arteries are also replaced every few weeks. Without protein, none of these vital processes could take place. So you can see why an adequate protein intake is vital.

Proteins are made of amino acids. The body uses twenty-six amino acids but can synthesize all but eight of them. Foods that contain all eight essential amino acids are called complete. High-protein foods include eggs, liver and other glandular meats, muscle meats, fish, poultry, milk and milk products, wheat germ, soy flour, and nuts.

Ten to 20 percent of your diet should come from proteins. Older people, however, may need to eat more protein because they don't digest, assimilate, and utilize their protein intake as well as younger people. If your diet includes a lot of legume products, such as navy beans, lima beans, or lentils, you may need extra protein because these foods aren't digested well by the body. Stress, too, increases the body's protein requirements.

CARBOHYDRATES

Carbohydrates come in two forms: sugars, which the body can use directly, and starches, which the body must break down before they can be assimilated. Nutritionists recommend that the bulk of our diet comes from complex carbohydrates, such as potatoes, legumes, and whole-grain bread. White-flour products, white rice, white sugar, and demineralized corn meal are all poor diet choices because they've been robbed of most of their normal vitamin and mineral content. For optimum nutrition, our carbohydrates should be as close to their natural form as possible, not denatured or processed.

The body requires only a small amount of fat in the diet, yet Americans consume a whopping 44 percent of their calories in the form of fat, which is a prime reason why we lead the world in heart disease and certain forms of cancer. In countries where fat intake is 20 percent or less, these diseases are rare. To prevent your arteries from getting clogged and to reduce your risk of colon and breast cancer, you should work to reduce the amount of fatty food in your diet. That means butter, whole milk, fatty meats, and fried foods should go on your taboo list. The biggest favor you can do for your body is to begin a lifelong low-fat diet today.

VITAMINS

Vitamins are organic substances that act as the spark to our internal combustion engine. Though vitamins are not foods and don't provide energy or build bulk or tissue, they are a vital part of our diets and must be replaced each day.

Vitamin supplementation is popular these days, but it's really a wrongheaded approach to nutrition. Vitamins should come from the foods we eat, not from drugstore shelves. If you want to take a daily vitamin that supplies roughly the Recommended Dietary Allowance (RDA) for vitamins and minerals, there's no harm in doing so. Megavitamin supplementation, however, can be dangerous, especially with the fat-soluble vitamins A and D, which can build up to toxic levels in the body if taken in excess. If you eat a varied diet, with regular and generous portions of vegetables, your vitamin needs should be taken care of.

MINERALS

Minerals, like vitamins, are an essential part of most of the body's processes. Calcium and phosphorus, for example, are needed for strong teeth and bones. Iron prevents anemia. Iodine helps regulate the body's metabolism. Minerals also play a part in the healing process; bruises, scratches, and cuts wouldn't heal without them. But even though minerals are a vital part of the diet, the actual amounts required are very small. A varied diet of fresh, unrefined food should give you all the minerals you require.

A high-fiber diet has been correlated with a reduced incidence of colon cancer. But don't overdo it. An excess of fiber can lead to diarrhea and mineral depletion.

RETESTING FOR FITNESS LEVELS

To keep your fitness program on track, you should periodically retest your fitness levels and compare your current readings with previous ones. If the step test shows that your cardiovascular fitness isn't what it should be, it could mean that you're not training intensely enough. The sit-up and push-up tests should also show improvements. Overall, how do you measure up? Is your weight and body fat where you want it to be? If not, readjust your exercise program. Everyone's metabolism is unique. If your exercise program isn't delivering the results you want, you shouldn't hesitate to tinker with it.

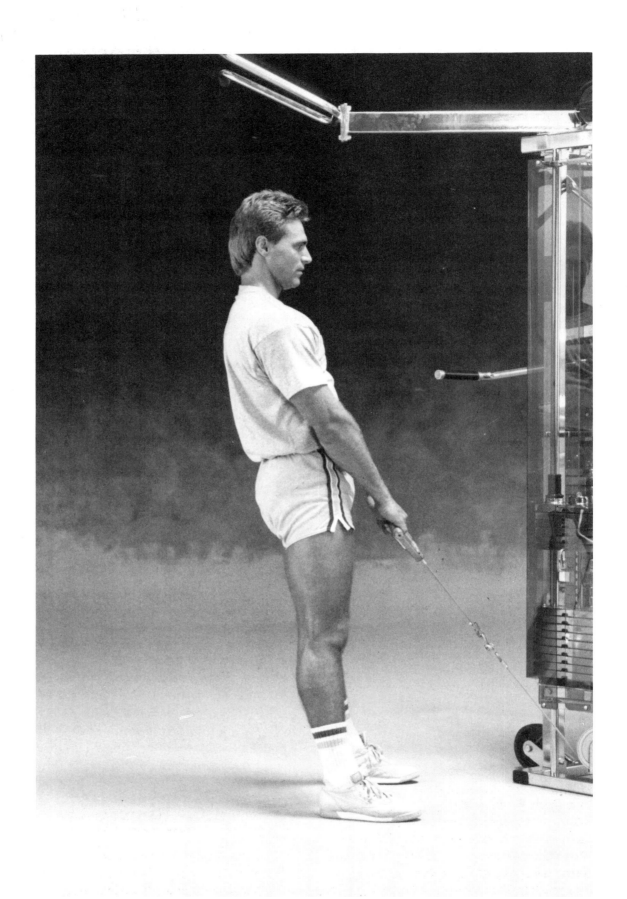

3

UNIVERSAL TRAINING PRINCIPLES AND FUNDAMENTALS

OVERLOADING MUSCLES

To get stronger, you have to work your muscles beyond their normal workload. The classic story told to illustrate this principle is about the ancient Greek Milo, who each day would raise his young calf above his head. After months of doing this, Milo was able to raise the animal, now a full-grown bull, above his head, which amazed the people of the town. The story probably is apocryphal. The principle, however, is true.

You must work your muscles beyond their normal limits to get results. You can do this in two ways: by lifting heavier weights or by lifting a lighter weight a greater number of times. The first method is associated with gains in strength, the second method with gains in muscle endurance.

But what exactly happens to muscles as a result of a weight-training program? Muscles that have been stressed undergo a variety of physiological changes. The muscle fibers themselves thicken. In addition, the connective tissue that binds the muscle fibers increases in amount and in tensile strength. The result is bigger muscles. This muscle growth is called hypertrophy. Its counterpart, atrophy, is the deterioration of muscle—exactly what happens to your muscles if you have to lie in bed for several weeks as a result of an injury or illness.

Muscle development depends on genetics. Few people can develop the musculature of world-class bodybuilders. Their genes just don't allow it. Women are sometimes afraid of developing huge, unsightly muscles, but the fact is that most women don't have enough testosterone, the male hormone, in their bloodstream to stimulate that kind of muscle growth, especially if they stick to light weights and endurance training.

PROGRESSIVE RESISTANCE

Universal workouts are based on the principle of progressive resistance, in which muscle strength is developed by doing exercises of gradually increasing resistance, such as pulling, pushing, or lifting weights. But the increases in strength aren't solely due to increases in muscle size. Part of the gain comes from increased muscle efficiency.

Muscles are made up of motor units, groups of muscle fibers that are stimulated by their own independent nerve supply. Stimuli will cause the muscle fibers in the motor unit to contract. Training increases the efficiency of the motor units within a given muscle function, allowing you to lift increasing amounts. As your muscles become developed through training, you'll be able to "recruit" more fibers and increase your strength and endurance.

Training improves the precision and economy of the motions in your workout. As training progresses, unnecessary static and dynamic muscular contractions are gradually eliminated as you learn to more completely relax the antagonistic muscle groups. The movement itself becomes more simple and automatic because reflexes replace, in part, the voluntary action, decreasing the energy required to perform a given motion. Naturally, beginners, who need to learn the particular skills, see the greatest improvements in coordination. Experienced athletes generally see less pronounced improvement in efficiency because they are already skilled in controlling their motions. However, athletes can still make tremendous gains through weight training, especially when training closely mirrors the activity the athlete is training for.

Increases in strength and efficiency are far more striking than the increases in muscle size. It's not unusual, for example, to increase the power of your muscles three times or more without a proportional increase in muscle volume. Unless you're a male with a genetic makeup for huge muscles, your strength gains are likely to be much more dramatic than the increase in your muscle size.

Circuit Training

Circuit training is a scientific arrangement of known and proven exercises designed to elicit maximum overall training effectiveness. Universal, by the nature and construction of its machines, has become the leader in this field.

The circuit programs outlined in this book are aimed at the development of all-around fitness, rather than at preparation for any particular game or sport. Each circuit offers varied activity and continuous challenge in a reasonable amount of time.

Universal's three major circuits—Antagonistic Muscle Circuit, Peripheral Heart Action Circuit, and Aerobic Super Circuit—are designed for improved strength, balanced conditioning, and aerobic endurance.

Circuit training has become one of the most popular forms of physical conditioning for a variety of reasons. Every individual can work at a rate and program that is most suitable for him or her. Weaker individuals can work independently, because the focus of the programs is on individual improvement. It doesn't matter that one person can bench press twice as much as another. What matters is that both are improving their performance by assessing their own progress and adjusting the intensity of the program accordingly.

Of course, the final results of circuit training depend on the kind of exercises you perform, the number of repetitions, the speed, the duration, the intensity of the contractions, and your genetic makeup. For some, the largest gains will be in strength—the power of each contraction. For others, it will be in endurance—the amount of work you're able to perform over a given period of time. But everyone benefits from working out.

HOW TO EXERCISE

First, some general guidelines. Your workout apparel should be loose and comfortable, allowing full freedom of motion.

To eat or not to eat? Don't wolf down a large meal before heading out to the gym. But a light snack eaten a few hours before your workout is certainly okay, and you may feel better if you have something in your stomach.

If you haven't worked out in a long time, your first workout is likely to leave you sore. Don't worry, this is a natural reaction for muscles that are not used to being stimulated. Part of the stiffness and soreness comes from lactic acid in the muscle tissues. As you become better trained—usually after two weeks—your body will become more efficient in dealing with lactic acid production, and soreness will cease to be a regular problem.

Generalized muscle soreness, however, shouldn't be confused with sharp, stabbing pains in a particular muscle region. Such pains indicate injury. You should stop working out those muscles until they are completely healed and the pain is completely gone.

Don't forget to breathe as you exercise. It's common to hold your breath while concentrating on a particularly difficult lift. Don't fall into that trap. Doing so can put a tremendous strain on your heart, which needs a constant supply of oxygen. Remember to exhale as you bring the weight up and inhale as you bring the weight down.

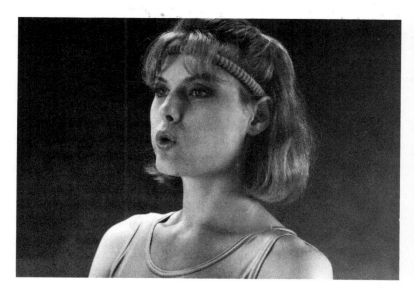

Exhale as you lift the weight

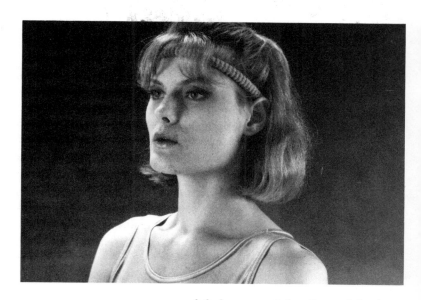

Inhale as you bring the weight down

INTENSITY, SPEED, AND FORM

To get results from a weight-training program, you must work hard enough to stimulate your muscles. But just how much is enough? Enough is that region between too much and too little. If you must struggle to complete the initial reps in the set, the weight is too heavy. Conversely, if you can do all the reps in the set without taxing yourself, the weight is too light. (Repetitions, or *reps*, are the number of times you perform a given exercise. If you do ten wrist curls, for example, you've performed ten reps. One series of reps constitutes a *set*.)

Beginners tend to overdo things. Don't try to become superhuman overnight. If you overextend yourself, a muscle tear or pull is likely. Don't try to lift more than you should just to impress yourself or other people in the gym. It doesn't matter that your friend can lift 125 pounds and you can lift only 75. What matters is that both of you are working hard enough to stimulate muscle growth. Health and fitness is a lifelong commitment. Don't push your body beyond what it's ready to handle. If you take things gradually and work out regularly, you'll get the improvements you're after.

Using proper form is just as important as using the proper weight. If the only way you can lift a weight is by relying on momentum or by contorting your body to gain added leverage, you should be using a lighter weight. Try to isolate the proper set of muscles for each exercise. That means no cheating—for example, no arching your back on the bench press. For full flexibility, you must perform the exercise through its full range of motion to make sure you fully extend and contract the muscle groups involved. Sometimes, however, you may not even be aware that your form is bad. So have an instructor make sure you're doing each exercise correctly. Habits, especially bad habits, are hard to break.

Execute each exercise smoothly and cleanly. Don't jerk the weight up or rely on momentum.

The counterpart of intensity is relaxation. Your body needs at least twenty-four hours to recover from the stress of exercise and form new muscle tissue, and without that rest, additional workouts will just break down your existing muscle tissue.

The other thing to watch out for is overtraining—exercising beyond your body's limits. You can overtrain even if you give yourself twenty-four hours between workouts. If your weight is down, your resting pulse is up, and you feel fatigued even after what would nor-

mally be adequate sleep, you're probably overtraining. The remedy is to take a few days off from your workout and relax. After some R&R, you should get your old energy level back. The cardinal rule in working out is to listen to your body's signals and respect them.

WEIGHT LOADS, REPS, SETS, CIRCUITS

What are your goals? To firm up? Gain strength? Lose weight? Increase muscle strength? Develop cardiorespiratory fitness or body build? Here are some general guidelines:

- For strength, size, and shape, train with five to seven repetitions, four to five sets for each exercise, with 70–90 percent of the single-rep maximum (the resistance at which one rep exhausts the muscle).
- For stamina and endurance, train with three sets of twelve to fifteen reps with 40–70 percent of your single-rep maximum.
- To lose weight, firm up, or increase cardiorespiratory fitness, train with three sets of fifteen to twenty reps with 40–50 percent of single-rep maximum, or do the Aerobic Super Circuit.
- For body building, we suggest a split routine. For example, on Monday and Thursday, exercise the chest, biceps, and abdominals; on Tuesday and Friday, the back, shoulders, and triceps; and on Wednesday and Saturday, the legs and abdominals. A seventy-two-hour recovery period between exercise sessions for each body part produces the best results. Each exercise should be performed in three to five sets of seven reps.

Specific weight-training circuits are described in Chapter 10. If you want to devise your own program, here's the direction the circuit should follow:

1. Bench or chest press.
2. Leg press or squats.
3. Lat pull.
4. Leg curl.
5. Shoulder press.
6. Hip flexor.
7. Triceps press-down.
8. Leg extension.
9. Arm curl.
10. Standing calf raise.
11. Upright row (low pulley).
12. Back arch (hyperextension).
13. Sit-ups.

Beginners will find that seven reps for most exercises is ideal for a strength program and twelve to fifteen for endurance programs. Sit-ups, hip flexor, and seated calf, however, should be done with fifteen reps. The weight used should be 40 to 80 percent of single-rep maximum, depending on whether you're a beginner or an advanced trainee. When you can complete the final reps in your program without difficulty, you should increase your weight load or adjust the number of reps or sets. In the early going, beginners may find themselves increasing the weights in their programs at a rapid rate. That's simply because an unconditioned body has more capacity for strength gains than one that is already near its peak.

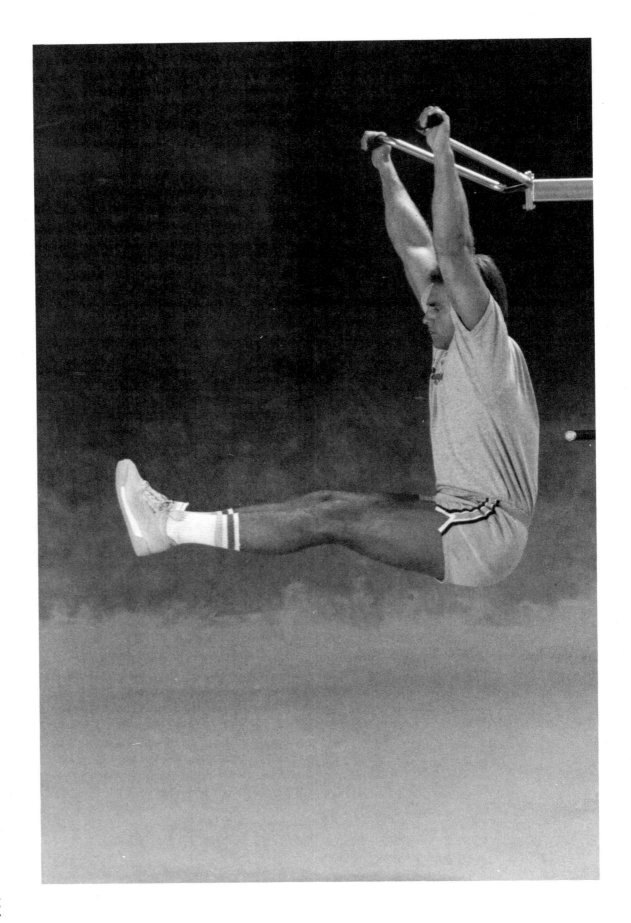

4

VARYING THE WORKOUT

TWELVE-WEEK WONDERS

We are cyclical beings. During sleep, we go through a number of predictable stages, from light sleep to heavy sleep, interspersed with periods of dreaming. Our respiration and heart rates follow regular patterns throughout the day. Women's menstrual periods roughly correlate with the lunar cycle. Scientists have just learned that morning heart attacks are associated with cyclical changes in the blood's clotting factors.

What does all this have to do with weight training? Everything! Our capacity for fitness gains has its own cycle, too—generally a cycle of twelve weeks. Thus, you'll usually see regular gains in strength and endurance for the first eight or ten weeks. But then, something strange starts to happen—the gains you've recorded drop off noticeably. Your overall performance becomes slack and lackluster, signaling that it's time for a change.

If you've been doing high reps with a low weight load, switch to low reps with a heavy weight load. Conversely, if you've been doing low reps with high weight load, you'll want to try the opposite. You can also vary the way you perform the exercises in your routine by using a different grip, or by changing your stance, or the position of your seat.

CHOOSING A GYM OR HEALTH CLUB

A large part of the success of your exercise program depends on where you work out. A club where people are dedicated to fitness is a much better motivator than a club where members are most concerned about making a date for Saturday night.

The first thing you should do is to make an appointment to see the gym. Most clubs can accommodate you if you just walk in off the street, but you're more likely to get a full review of the facilities if the club personnel know in advance that you're coming. Make your appointment for the same time that you'd be using the gym. Many clubs are like Grand Central Station after five o'clock, and there are few things more frustrating than having to wait in line for the next machine in your circuit because of overcrowding. You want to see if you're going to have to struggle against crowds if you decide to join. But be real-

istic. Don't expect the club to be deserted between 5:00 P.M. and 7:00 P.M.— prime workout hours. Be sure to ask about the club's hours. Maybe you can beat the crowds by scheduling an early-morning or lunchtime workout.

The first thing to do is to check out the equipment itself. Does it look well-maintained? Does it work smoothly or does it have a tendency to stick because of misaligned parts? Is it clean? Sweaty bodies can make the equipment's padding a breeding ground for bacteria if it is not cleaned regularly. How about the locker rooms? Are they clean? Are there enough shower stalls? How is the club's climate control? The temperature should be cool but not so cold that you're uncomfortable. These questions may seem nitpicky, but they're not. The main reason people drop out of their workout program is not the injuries, but lack of motivation. A run-down, grungy health club can quickly make you wonder why you ever started working out in the first place.

Next check out the instructors' credentials. Do they have a background in sports and fitness? Give extra points to clubs whose instructors have completed the Universal Fitness Institute's four-day certification program. After all, the people who best know how to use Universal equipment are the people who created it. This course gives instructors the best advice available on:

- Screening individuals for medical risk.
- Conducting initial testing to determine each person's current level of fitness.
- Establishing realistic fitness goals.
- Recommending the proper exercises.
- Motivating and instructing creatively.

You'll do best at a club whose instructors have the knowledge to help you make maximum gains with minimal chance for injury. Stay away from clubs whose instructors' main qualifications are that they have nice smiles and look good in gym suits.

Last, you want to know about the club's finances. How long has it been around? If it folds (or if you move), can you transfer your membership to another club? Try to talk to some of the club members privately to get the real scoop on the club. Are people generally satisfied with the club or are real improvements needed? How much is the basic membership? Often, special deals are available, so ask the club's instructors and the club members about them.

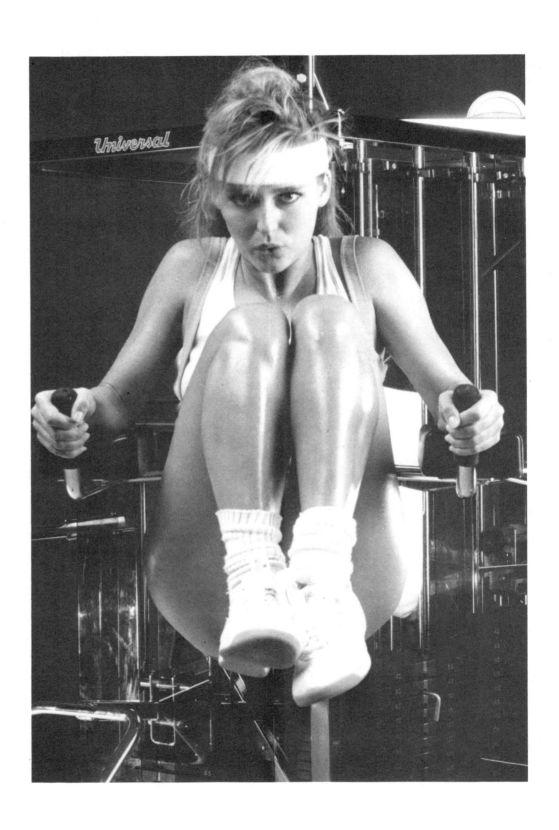

5

Warming Up

Warm-Up

Muscles function better warm than cold. A warm-up brings more oxygen-rich blood to the muscles by increasing your heart and respiratory rates and by dilating your blood vessels. The warm-up also prepares your heart and lungs for the demands you're going to place on them. The warm-up, in short, is a necessary prelude to the stretching phase and your body's rehearsal for the actual workout. So before you start stretching your muscles, you should either jog slowly in place, walk briskly on a treadmill, or pedal comfortably on a stationary bike. After you've worked up a light sweat (allow five to ten minutes), you're ready to start stretching.

Stretching

In the past, bouncing, or ballistic, stretches were the norm. We now know that static stretches are a safer way to stretch muscles. Our muscles and tendons are like rubber bands. If you quickly stretch a cold muscle, you risk injury, because the momentum of the movement can easily take your muscles beyond their normal limits. The result: Your muscle snaps just like a rubber band would if stretched beyond its limits.

Static stretching, on the other hand, is much safer and just as effective as ballistic stretching, because body segments are moved slowly through their range of motion until they can go no further, and that position is held for ten to thirty seconds and then relaxed. This motion is repeated several times. If you want an in-depth book on the subject, take a look at Bob Anderson's *Stretching* (Shelter Publications).

Your flexibility level, just like your strength and endurance levels, is unique. Respect your body's limits. Don't use the warm-up as a competitive phase. The only thing you should be competing with is your past performance. Work slowly toward improving your body's flexibility. The gains will come if you give them time.

Here are some stretches that will help elongate most of the muscles in your body:

Hamstring Stretch. While standing erect, cross one foot over the other. Keep the heel of the crossed leg up (to keep the pelvis straight). Reach down toward the ground until you feel a slight pull in the back of your leg. Hold this position for fifteen to thirty seconds. One rep.

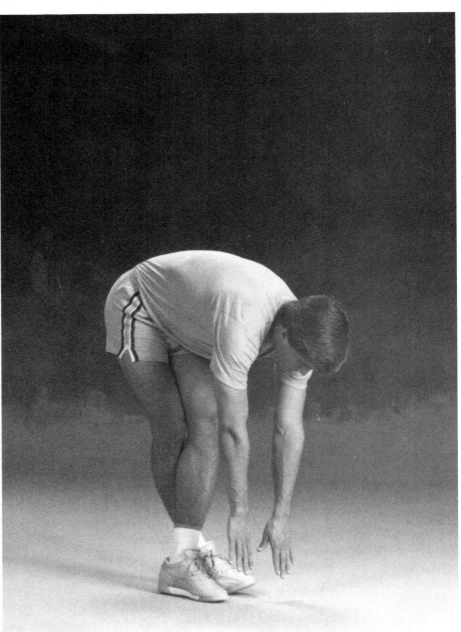

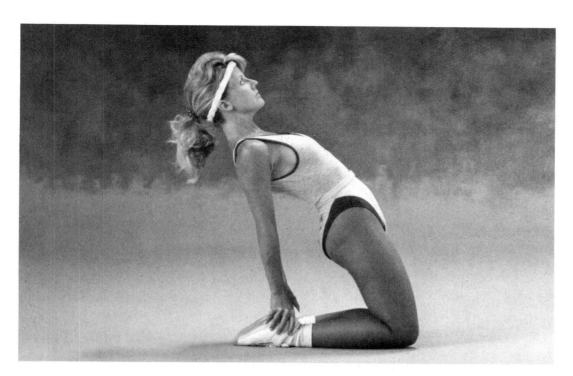

Quadriceps Stretch. Kneel with your toes pointed away from your body. Lean back and place your hands on the heels of your feet, raising your pelvis up and out. Let your head drop back. You should feel the stretch in the quadriceps, the muscles on the front of your thighs. Hold this position for fifteen to thirty seconds. One rep.

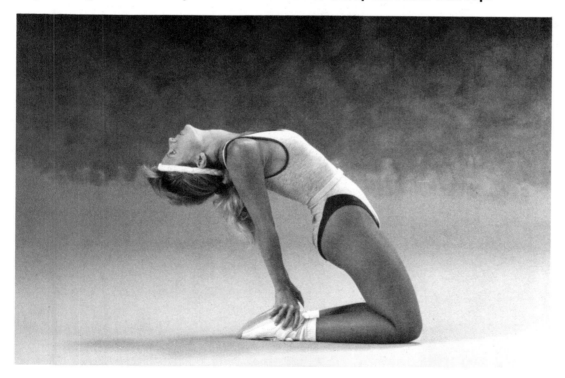

Good Morning Stretch. With your knees bent, place the tips of your fingers on the ground. Stand up, then rise on the tips of your toes with your hands extended straight over your head. One rep.

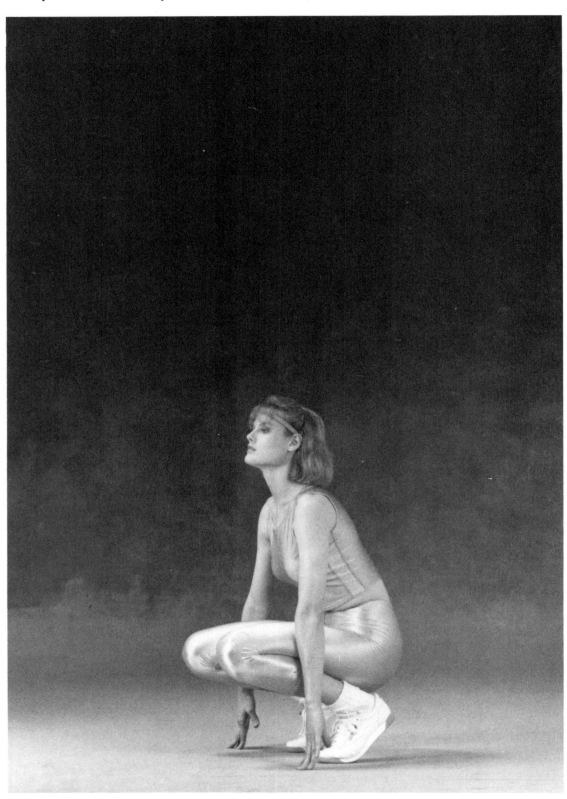

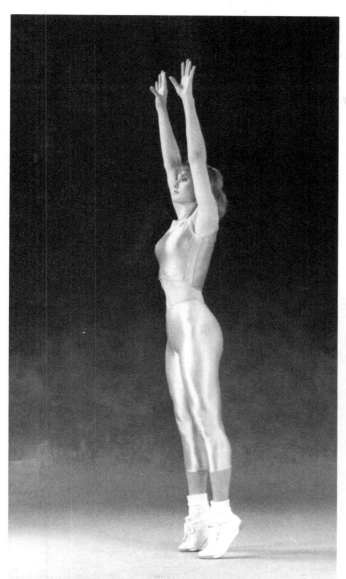

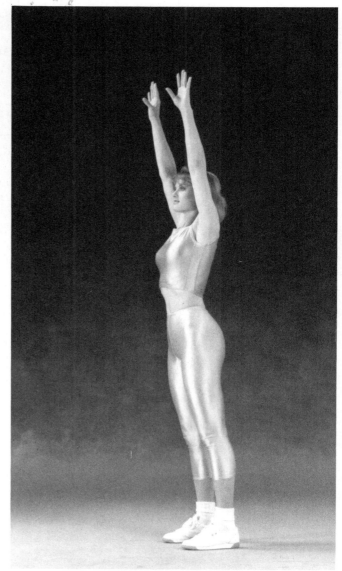

Achilles Stretch. **While standing, place the palms of your hands on a wall in front of you and move your feet as far as possible away from the wall. While on your toes, stretch your heels toward the floor and hold the position for ten to twenty seconds. One rep.**

Seated Toe Touch. **This stretch is for the back and hamstrings. Sit on the floor with your legs extended in front of you and your toes pointed out. Slowly slide your hands down your legs until you feel the stretch. Try to grasp your ankles and slowly pull until your head approaches your legs. Hold the position for ten to twenty-five seconds. One rep.**

Knee Pull. **This stretch is for your trunk and thighs. Sitting on the floor with the balls of your feet together, pull one leg toward your chest and hold for a count of five. Repeat with the opposite leg. Do seven to eight times for each leg.**

Groin Stretch. **While sitting on the floor, place the balls of the feet together and pull the toes toward your groin. Stretch forward while pressing down on the knees with your elbows. Hold the position for ten to twenty seconds. One rep.**

Standing Quad Stretch. **While standing, reach back and grab the front of your ankle, bending your knee. Pull your heel back as far as possible toward your buttocks. Hold position for fifteen seconds. One rep.**

Push-Up with Back Arch. **Bend forward, placing your hands on the floor about three to four feet from your feet. Arch your back and raise your head and shoulders. Extend your arms until straight and perform a push-up.**

Neck Circles. **Standing with your feet apart, gently roll head in a full circle, first in one direction, then in the other. Do three complete circles in each direction.**

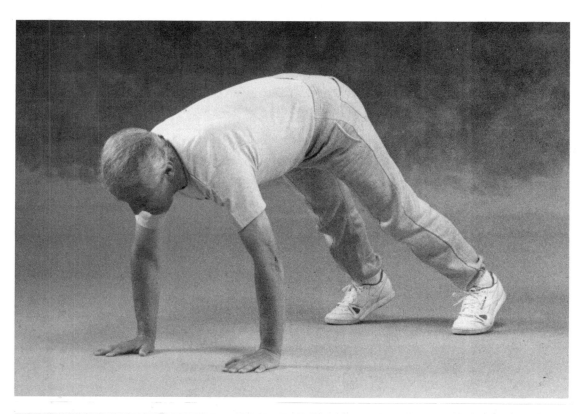

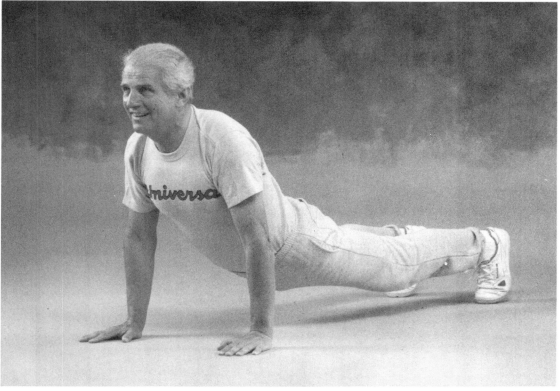

Caterpillar Push-Up. **With your trunk parallel to the floor and your legs straight, place your palms and toes flat on the ground. Your buttocks should be higher than your head. Bring your pelvis down and forward and your head up.**

Side Bender. While standing, place your left hand on your left hip and place the right hand over your head. Slowly bend to the left, toward the hand on the hip. Stretch gently. Repeat five times on each side.

Low-Back Trunk Twister. Bend forward at the waist with your legs spread slightly wider than shoulder width. Bend your arms at the elbow to form right angles, keeping your forearms parallel to the ground. With a wide sweeping motion, move your arms left and right, rotating the trunk and stretching in each direction while holding your head stationary. Repeat twenty to twenty-five times.

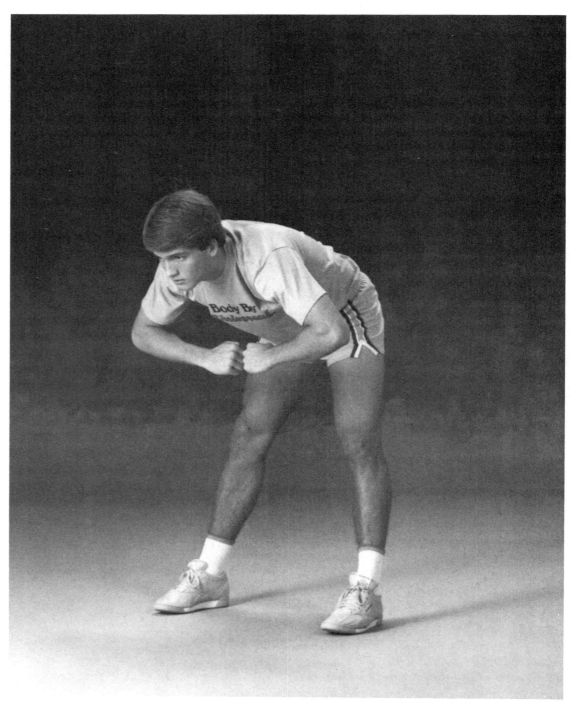

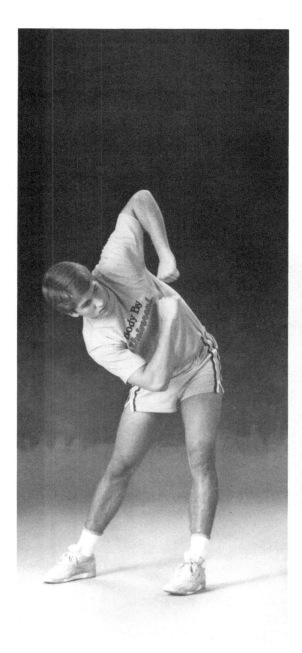

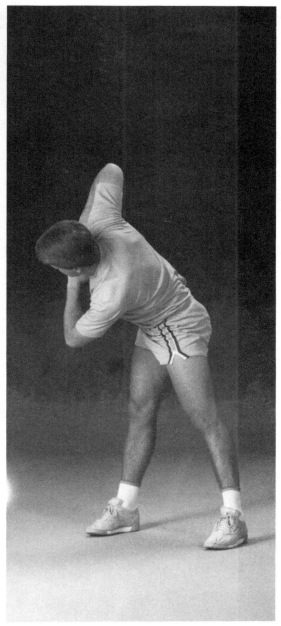

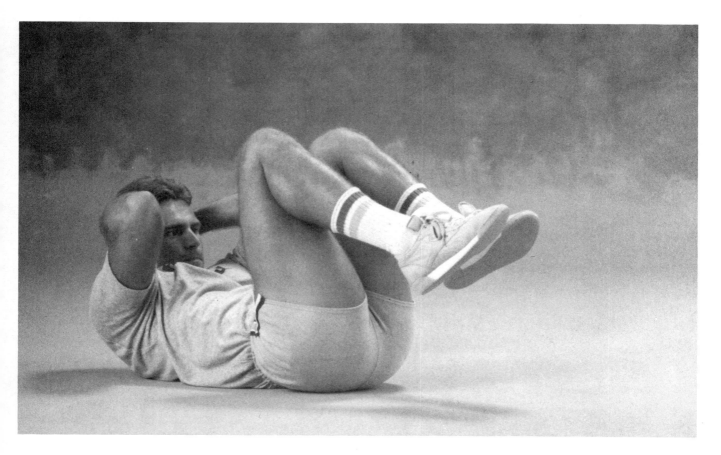

Abdominal Twister. Lying with your back on the floor, put your hands behind your head, pull your knees toward your chest, and raise your head toward your knees until your body is in a cradle position. (Be careful not to pull on your head.) Touch your right elbow to your left knee, then your left elbow to your right knee. Alternate, maintaining control. Build up to approximately fifty repetitions.

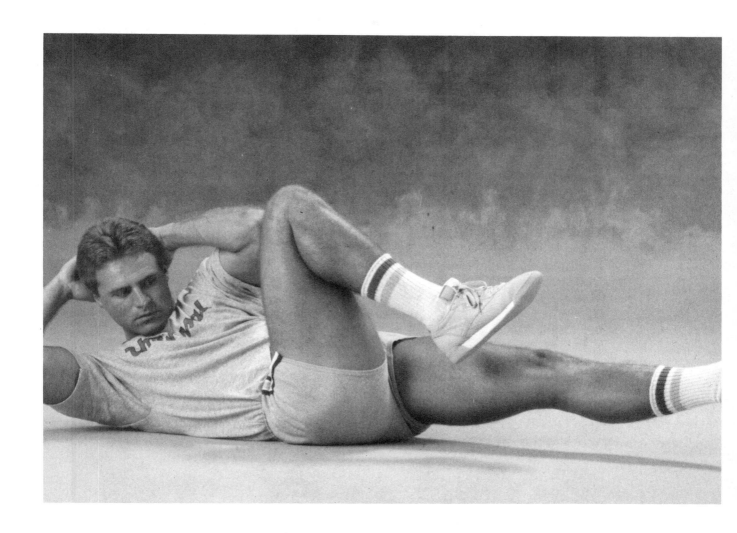

COOL-DOWN

After you've finished your workout, go through your stretching program again. You'll find that your fully warmed muscles are much more pliable and stretch easily. This postworkout stretching is a good way to prevent injury and ward off the stiffness that often accompanies muscular exertion.

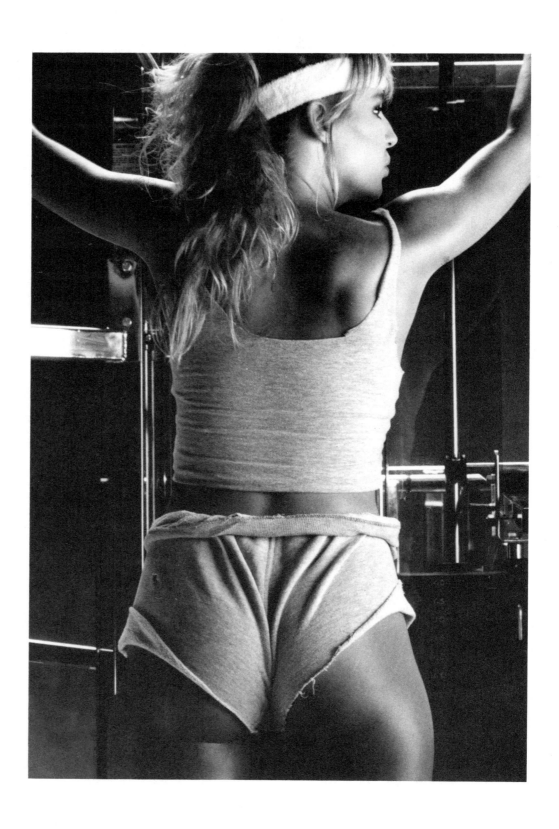

6

TRAINING AND BUILDING THE LEGS AND HIPS

The legs and hips are too often an overlooked area of the body in terms of overall physical fitness. Strong legs and a strong torso are crucial in most sports, from basketball and baseball, to soccer football and tennis. Well conditioned legs are also an important part of an attractive appearance. No one wants to be stuck with saddle-bags and cellulite. And of course a well conditioned lower body plays a fundamental role in locomotion, which is of great concern to older exercisers. Once the muscle tone and strength of the hips and lower legs is gone, it is gone forever. Take special care not to pass over these important muscle groups.

LEG PRESS EXERCISES

Primary muscle group affected: quadriceps.

General instructions: Sit up straight with your lower back against the back of the seat station. Grasp the handles on the side of the chair to keep from sliding.

REGULAR LEG PRESS

Lean back into the seat and drive the weight up, extending your legs fully at the knee joint. Exhale as you push the weights up. Then return your feet to the starting position, carefully controlling the weights. Don't let the weights touch the stack when doing multiple repetitions.

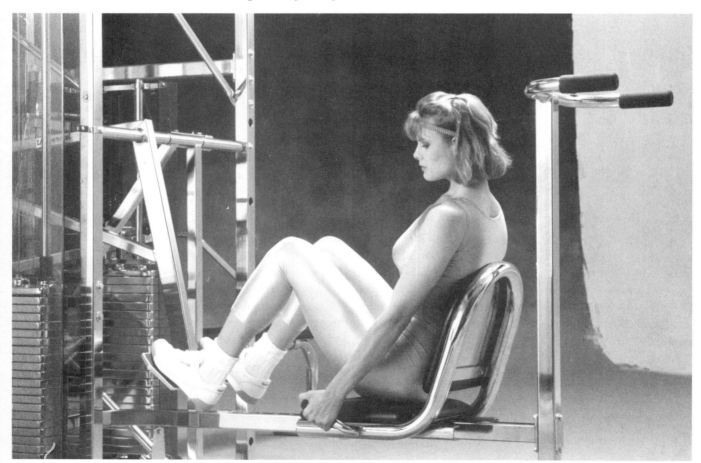

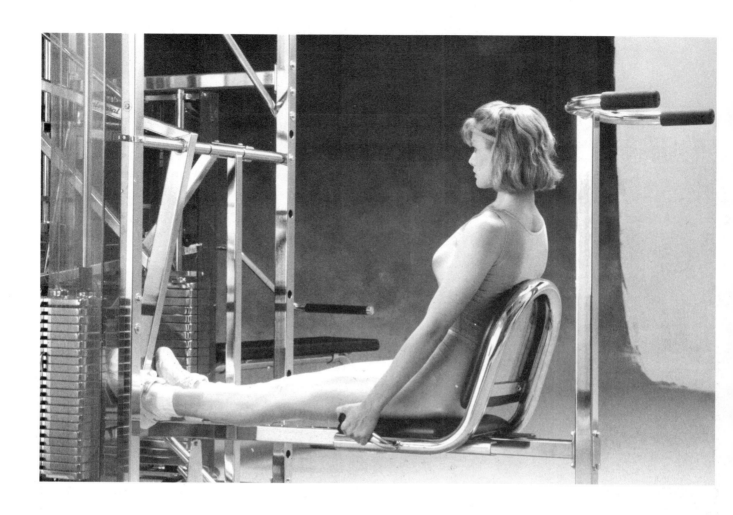

SINGLE LEG PRESS (Optional)

If one of your legs is weaker than the other, you can do additional repetitions of
the regular leg press using just the weaker leg.

CALF, ANKLE, ARCH PRESS

Place the balls of your feet on the pedals and press the weights back and forth with quick extension movements. Try to extend your feet as far as possible when pressing with your toes, and let your feet come back as far as possible in the return phase (without touching or resting on the stack). There are three possible toe positions: straight ahead, toes out, and toes in.

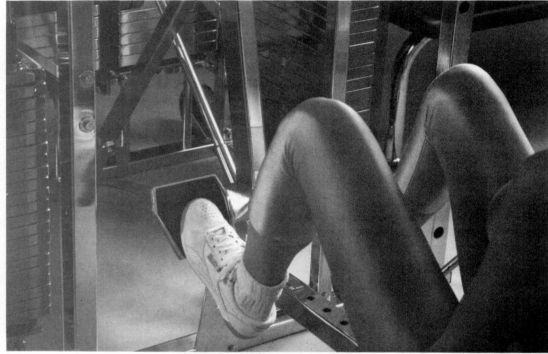

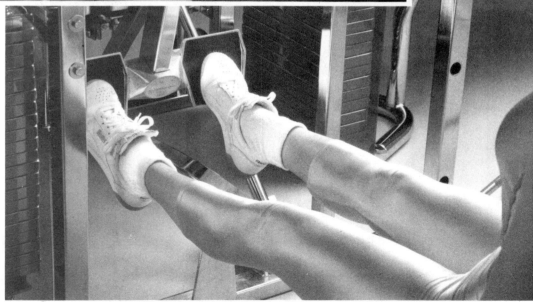

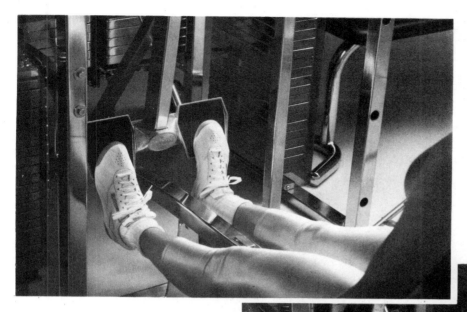

Above, toes straight ahead. Right, toes out. Below, toes in.

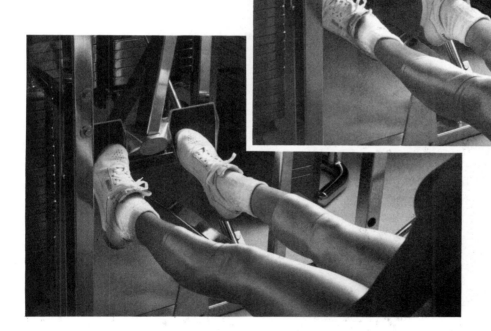

SINGLE CALF EXTENSION (Optional)

If one of your calves is weaker than the other, you can do additional repetitions for the calf, ankle, arch press using just the weaker leg.

Sprinter Kick Back

Muscle
groups
affected:

buttocks,
hamstrings,
and
quadriceps.

Facing away from the machine, straddle the chair, resting your hands on the back of the seat. Lean over and bring your head down, dropping your hips. Place one foot against the pedal and keep the supporting leg straight. Press back with the first leg against the weight, extending the motion through your hip.

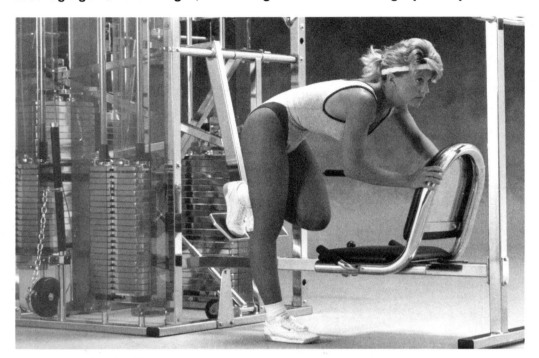

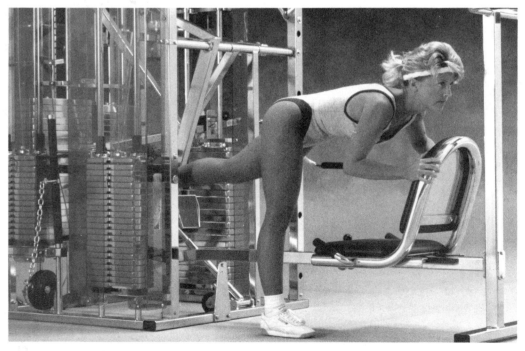

ABDOMINAL BOARD EXERCISES

SIDE LEG RAISES

Place the board at a thirty-degree angle. Lie on the board on your side with your head toward the rollers. Grasp the side of the board with one hand, with your other arm cushioning your head. Your legs should be straight. Lift your top leg, leading with your heel, as high as possible, then lower it slowly to the starting position. Repeat the exercise to complete the set. Then turn on your other side and repeat the set.

Muscle groups affected:

abductor muscles of the upper leg.

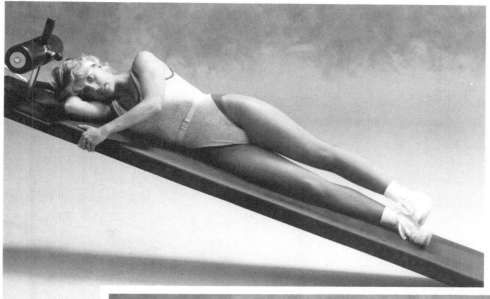

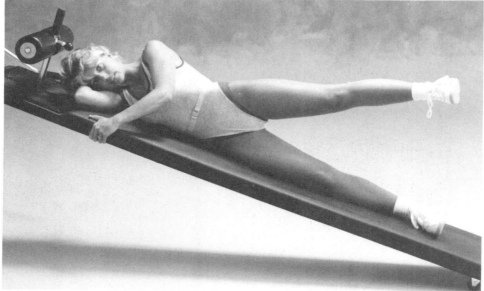

THIGH AND KNEE MACHINE EXERCISES

The knee is controlled by the quadriceps and hamstrings working in opposition to each other. Leg extensions develop the quadriceps; leg curls develop the hamstrings. The stronger these muscles, the stronger your legs and knees will be. The hamstrings and quadriceps should be roughly equal in strength.

DOUBLE LEG EXTENSION

Muscle groups affected:

quadriceps, and thigh.

Sit upright on the leg extension table, placing the tops of your feet under the bottom of the rollers. Reach back and hold on to the table with your hands. Lock your ankles but don't point your toes. Lift both legs together. At the completion of the extension, flex both thighs hard. Lower the weight under control, taking care not to let the weight touch or rest on the stack. Repeat.

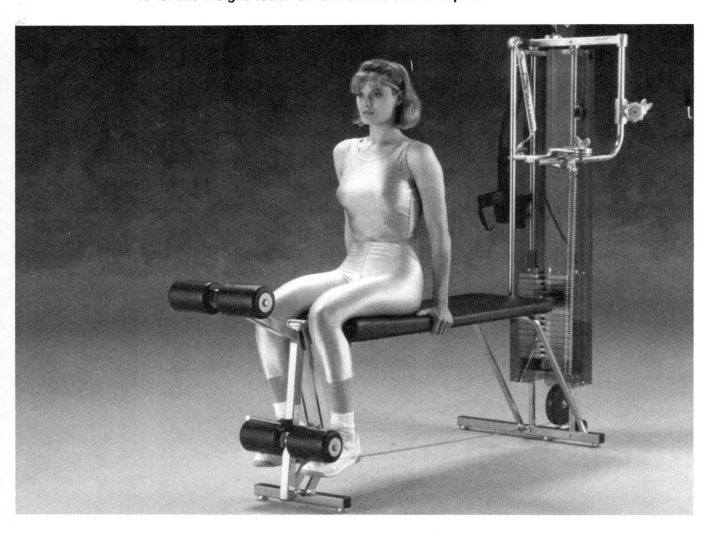

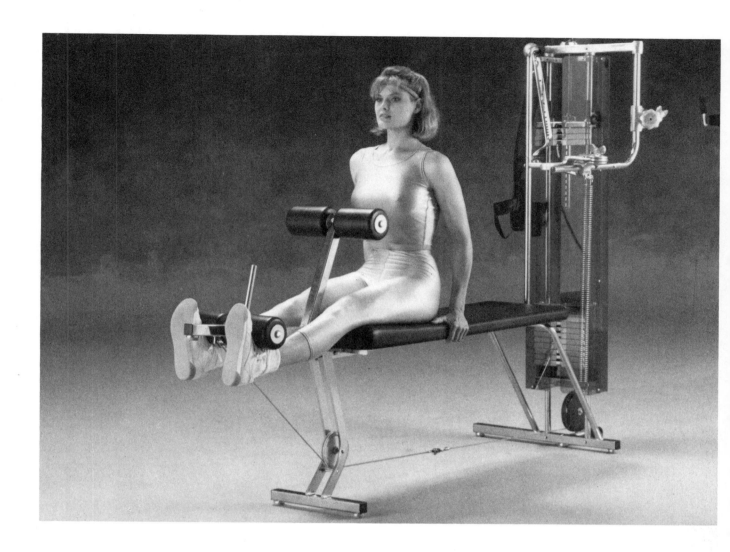

Single Leg Extension

Sit upright on the bench, placing the tops of your feet under the bottom of the rollers. Reach back and hold on to the bench with your hands. Lift one leg. At the completion of the extension flex your thigh hard. Lower the weight under control to the starting position and repeat the exercise using the other leg. Because one leg is usually dominant over (stronger than) the other, this is the best way to exercise these muscles if you want to build both legs equally, or concentrate on building up an injured leg.

Muscle groups affected:

quadriceps, thigh, and knee tendon.

DOUBLE LEG CURL

Lie on your stomach on the bench. Place your heels under the rollers with your knees in line with the pivot point or pin. Keep your hips and chest down. Hold on to the legs of the bench with your hands. Pull your heels as far as possible toward your hips. (Note: if your hips rise, you're using too much weight.) Lower the weight slowly to its starting point, taking care not to let the weight touch the stack, and repeat the exercise.

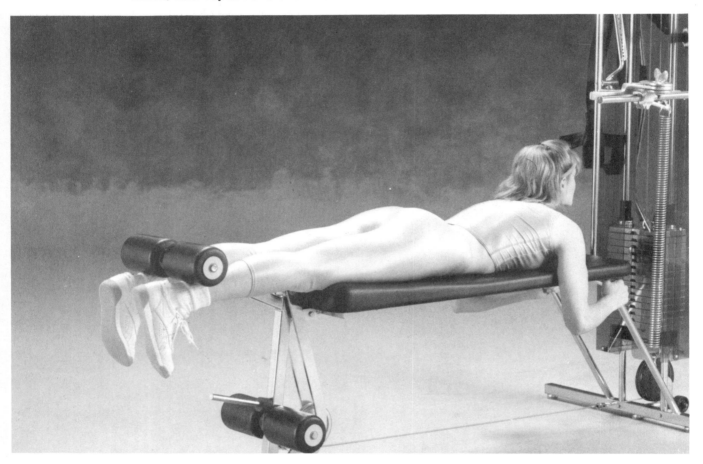

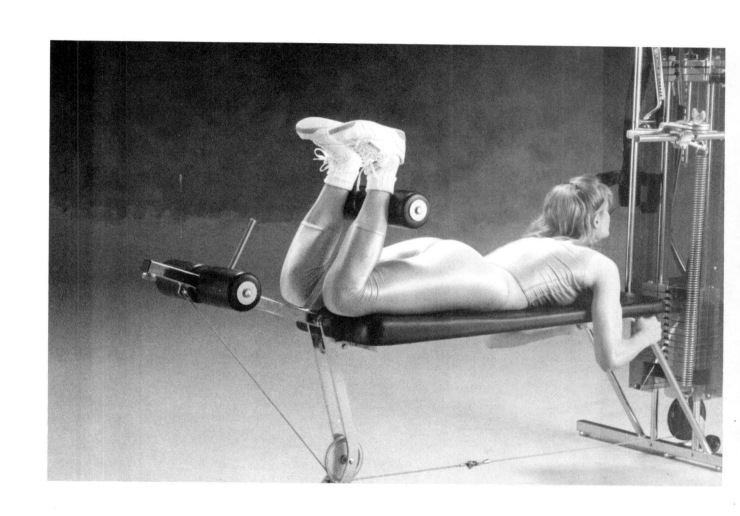

CALF RAISE

Place a block of wood (at least three inches high) on the floor in line with the handles. Stand facing the machine with your shoulders over the handles of the chest press and the balls of your feet on the edge of the block. To develop your inner and outer muscles equally, keep your feet straight ahead. To develop the inside of your muscles, turn your feet out. To develop the outside of your muscles, turn your feet in. Drive the weight up as far as possible, keeping your knees slightly locked. Bring the weight down slowly and touch your heels to the floor.

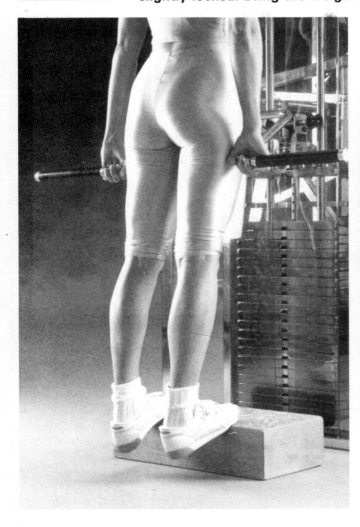

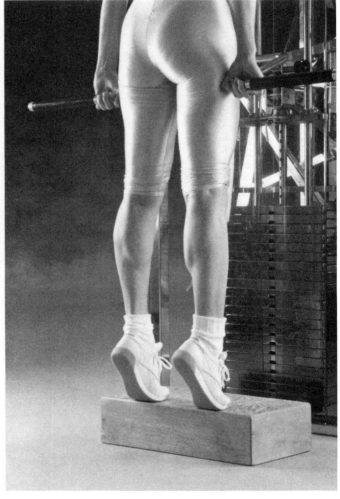

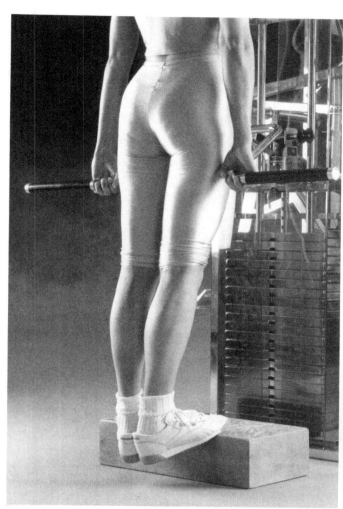

Calf Raise—feet straight ahead

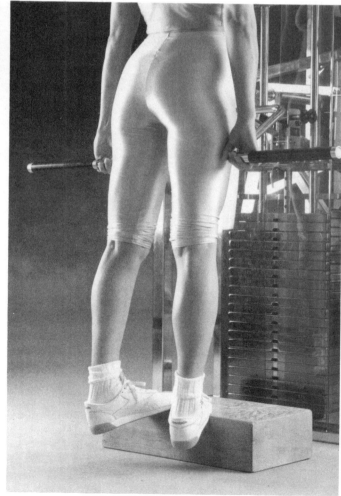

Calf Raise—feet turned in

LEG PRESS

Muscle
groups
affected:

quadriceps,
hip flexors,
buttocks.

Lie on the floor and place your feet under the handles of the chest press. Drive your legs up until they are fully extended. Lower slowly. Repeat.

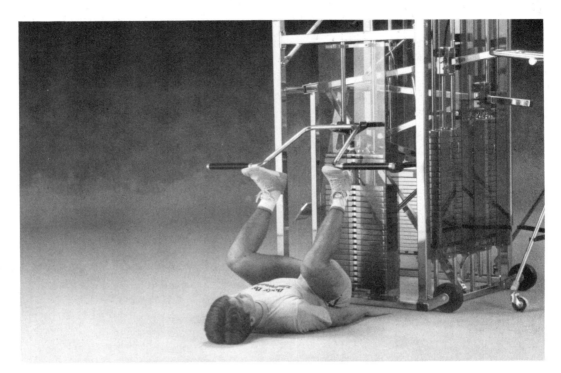

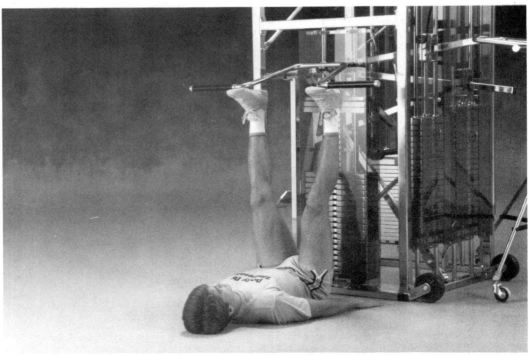

ADDUCTOR KICK (Using the Ankle Strap)

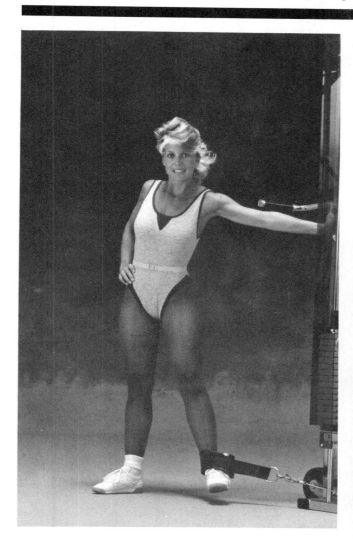

Place the ankle strap around the ankle closest to the machine. Stand next to the machine with your legs far apart. Grip the frame and place your other hand on your hip. Pull your inside leg across the other leg and return to your starting position with control. Repeat the exercise by turning the other way and using the other leg.

Muscle groups affected:

adductor muscles of the hip.

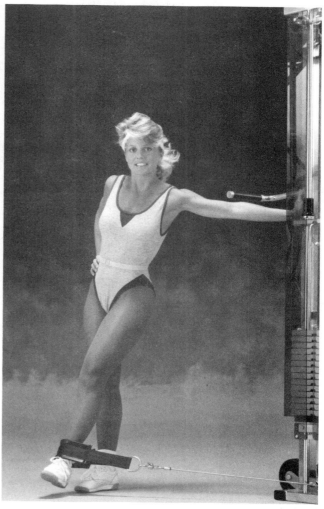

ABDUCTOR KICK (Using the Ankle Strap)

Muscle group affected:

abductor muscles of the upper outside leg.

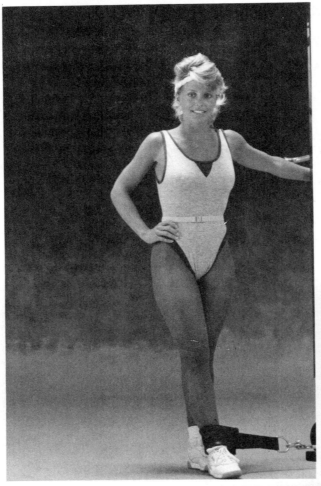

Place the ankle strap around the ankle farthest from the machine. Stand with the leg with the ankle strap on it in front of the other leg. Grip the frame and place your other hand on your hip. Kick or raise your far leg to the side, up and out, leading with the heel, and then return with control. Repeat the exercise by turning the other way and using the other leg.

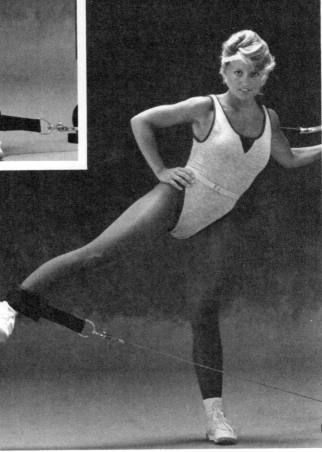

BACK HIP EXTENSION
(Using the Ankle Strap)

Place the ankle strap around one ankle. Stand erect facing the machine. Grip the frame and place your other hand on your hip. Kick your leg straight back at the hip joint as far as possible, keeping your knee straight. Return to the starting position with control. Repeat the exercise using the other leg.

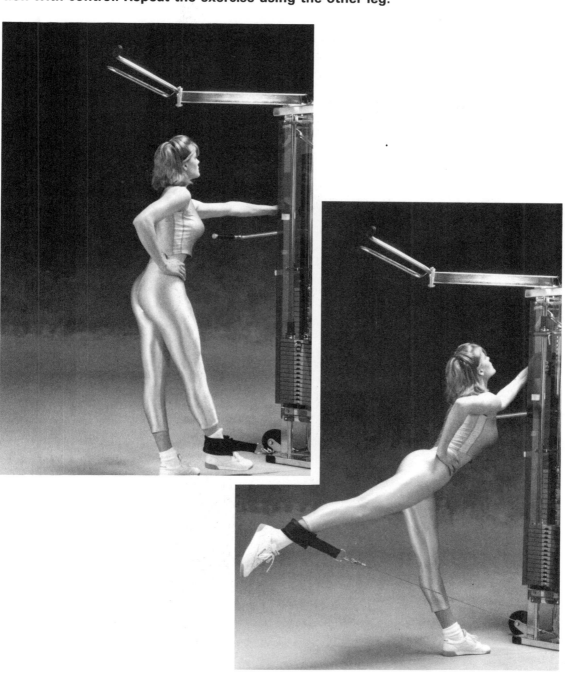

HIP FLEXOR

Place the ankle strap around one ankle. Lie on your back on the floor, your feet toward the machine. Pull your knee to your chest, then return to your starting position. Repeat the exercise using the other leg.

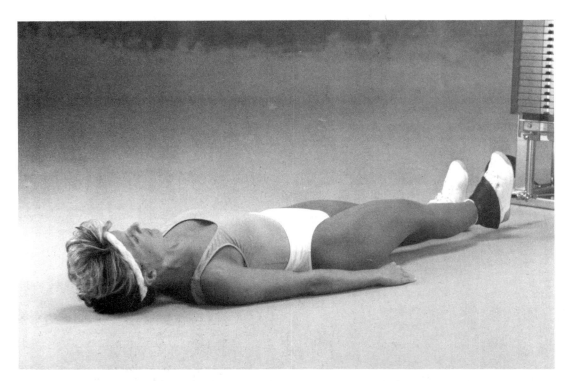

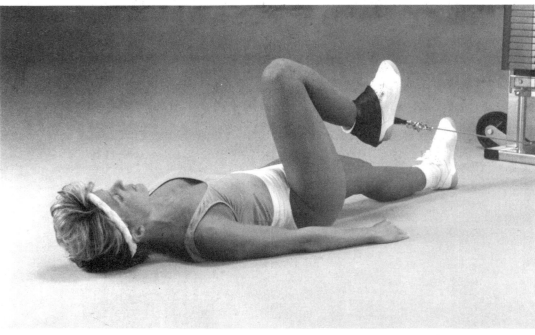

7

TRAINING AND BUILDING THE UPPER TORSO, ARMS, AND NECK

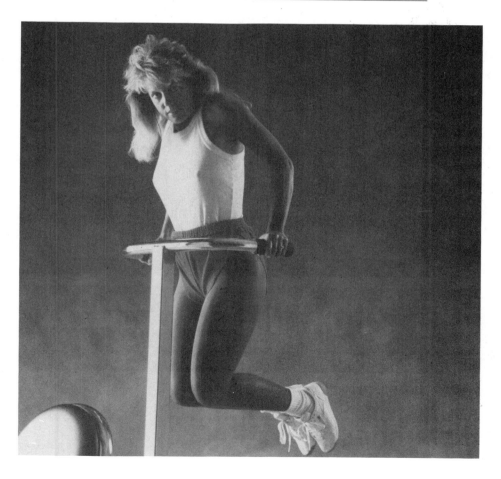

CHEST PRESS EXERCISES

Primary muscle groups affected: pectorals [chest], deltoids [shoulder], triceps.

General instructions: Compensate for right- or left-hand dominance by moving your weaker hand out one-half inch to three-quarters of an inch further on the handles than your stronger hand.

BENCH PRESS (Chest Press)

Muscle groups affected:

pectorals, deltoids, triceps.

Lie on the bench with your head toward the machine and your feet on the floor. Keep your elbows in close to your sides. The bend of the handles should be above your chest. Press the weight up, exhaling sharply. Inhale while returning the weight as far as possible without touching the remaining stack. The weight should be lowered with control. Repeat.

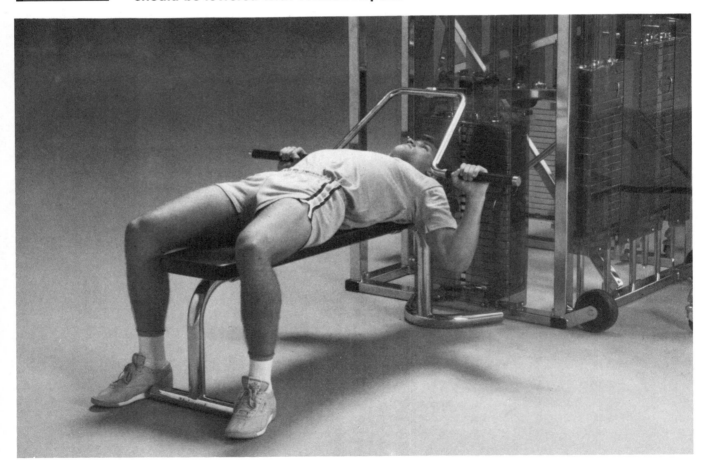

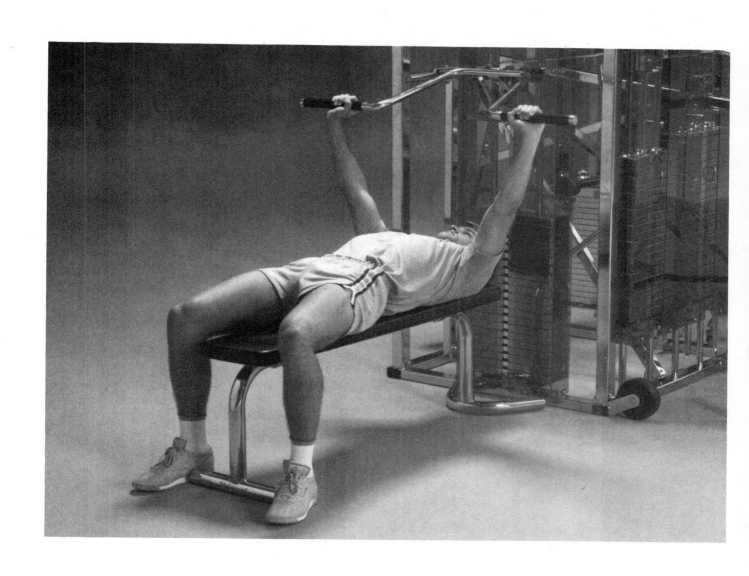

SHOULDER SHRUG

Muscle groups affected:

Upper back muscles, specifically the trapezius [upper back], rhomboids, and deltoids.

Stand facing the machine and grasp the handles, using a narrow or close grip. Shrug your shoulders by lifting them toward your ears and rotating them backward. Inhale and lift your sternum. Now exhale and return the weight almost to the starting position, using control. Repeat.

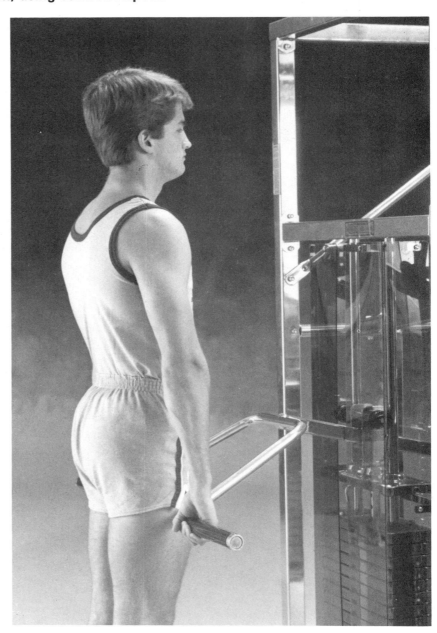

Starting position

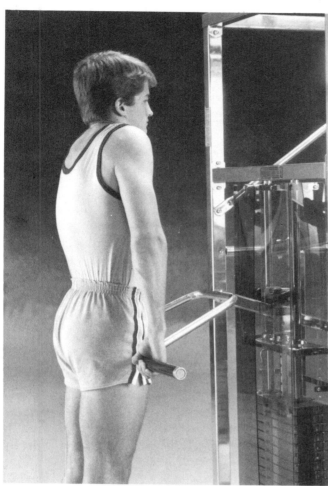

Lift your shoulders toward your ears in a shrug, then rotate your shoulders backward

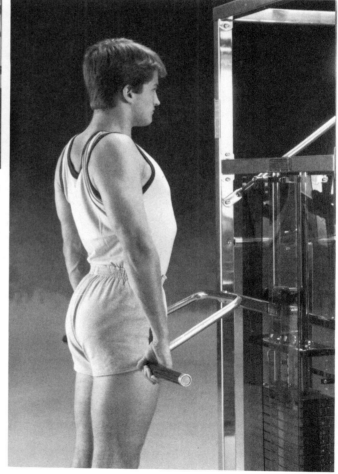

Inhale and lift your sternum

Leg Raise and Chest Press Combination

Lie flat on the bench with your head toward the machine and your legs extended straight out. Simultaneously press the weight up and raise your legs over your head, exhaling as you do so. Be sure to keep your legs straight. Lower the weight and your legs and repeat.

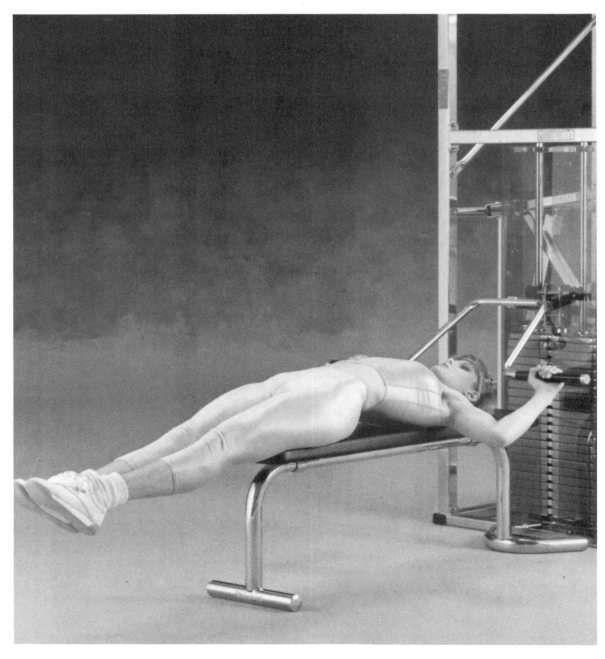

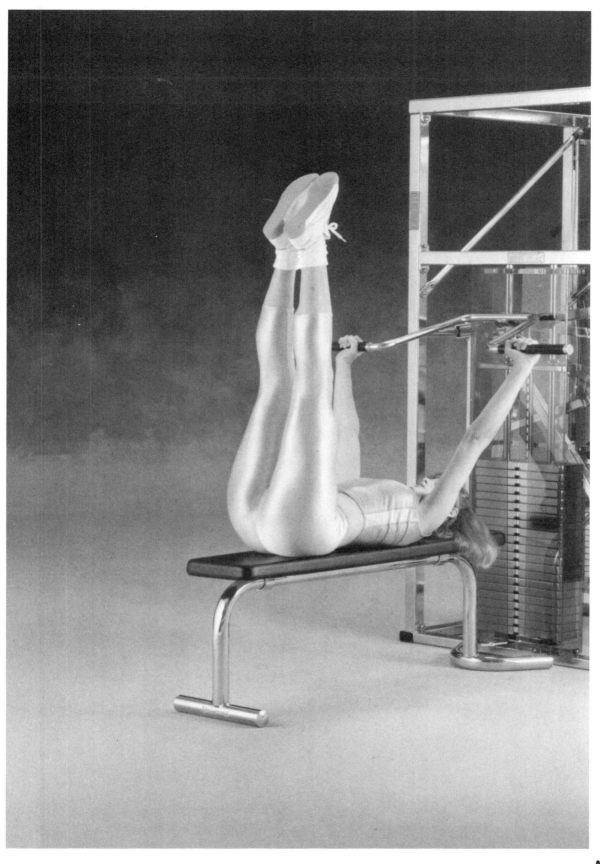

SINGLE-ARM SIDE CHEST PRESS

Muscle groups affected:

pectorals, deltoids, and triceps.

Turn the bench sideways to the machine. Lie on the bench; the handle should be even with or below chest level. (You may elevate the bench with a block of wood if necessary.) Exhale as you push the weight up, using one arm to perform the press. Lower the weight slowly. Repeat.

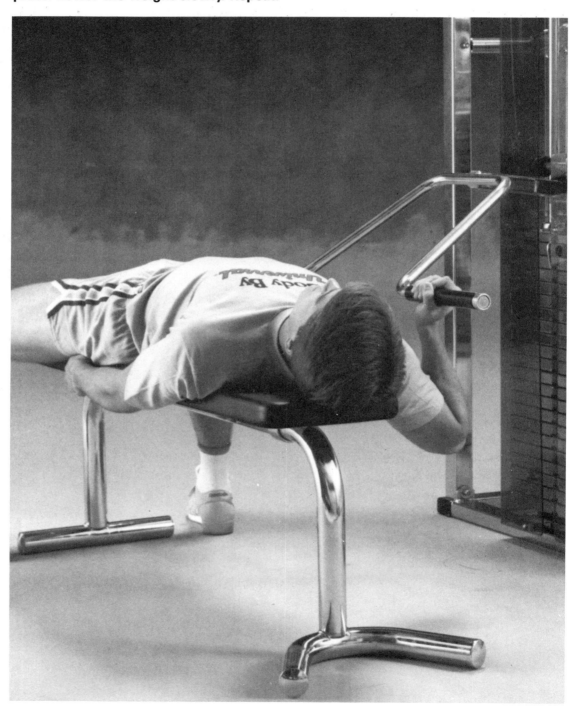

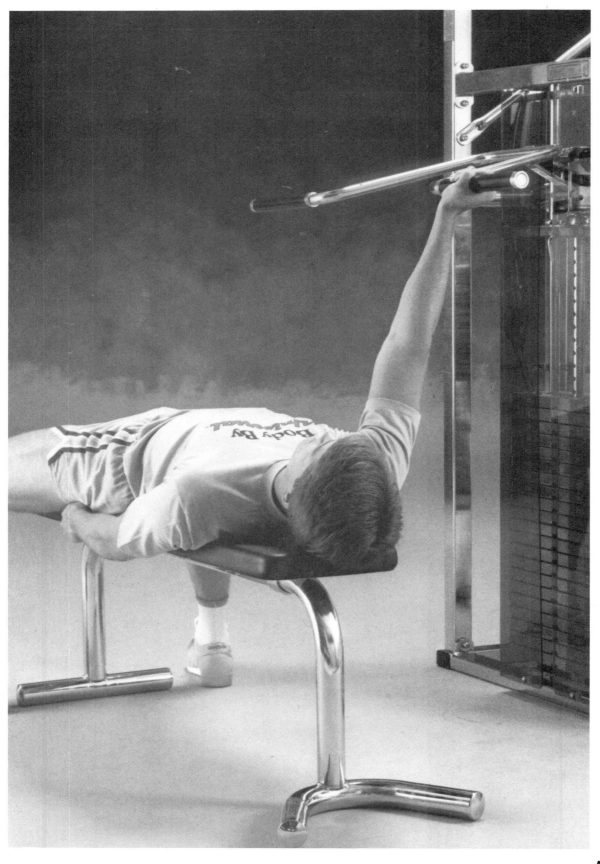

DEAD LIFT (Advanced Exercise)

Stand on a box or bench, facing the machine. Keep your head up and your back flat. Bend and grasp the handles, keeping your arms straight. Lift the weight, first using your legs and then your back, until you are back to a standing position. Inhale high in your chest. While exhaling, lower the weight to the starting position, exhaling at the bottom position. Repeat.

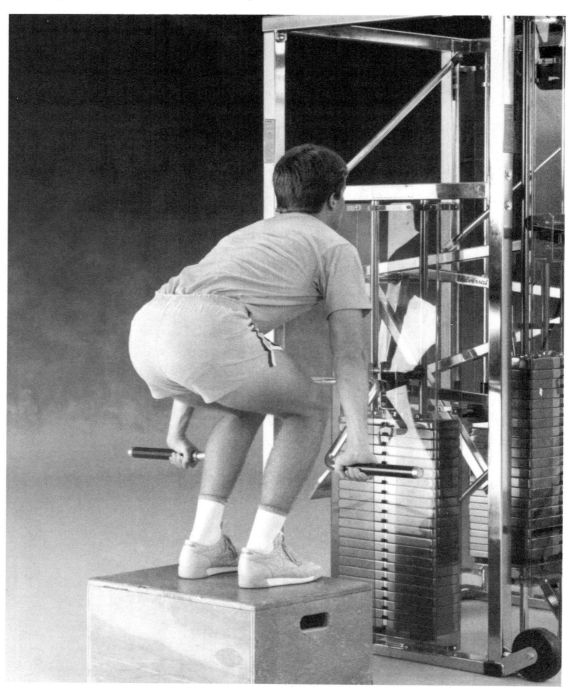

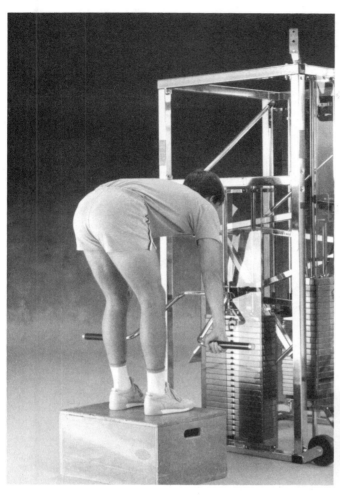

Left, starting position. Above, lift the weight first with your legs. Right, then lift the weight with your back.

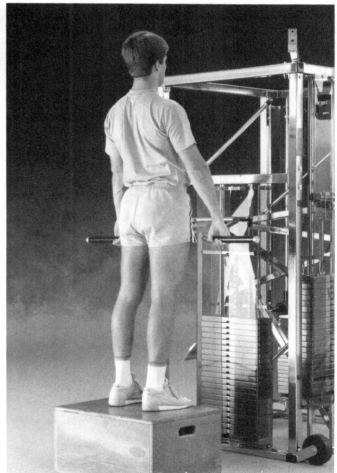

SHOULDER PRESS EXERCISES

Primary muscle groups affected: deltoids, triceps, and trapezius (upper back).

FORWARD SHOULDER PRESS

Muscle groups affected:

deltoids, triceps.

Sit facing the machine with your shoulders almost touching the handles. Place your feet inside the rungs of the stool to prevent yourself from pushing with your legs. You may use either a wide or a close grip. Exhale as you push the weight up; inhale coming down. To keep your back flat, watch the weight throughout the press. Do not allow the weight to touch the stack when lowering it to the starting position. Repeat.

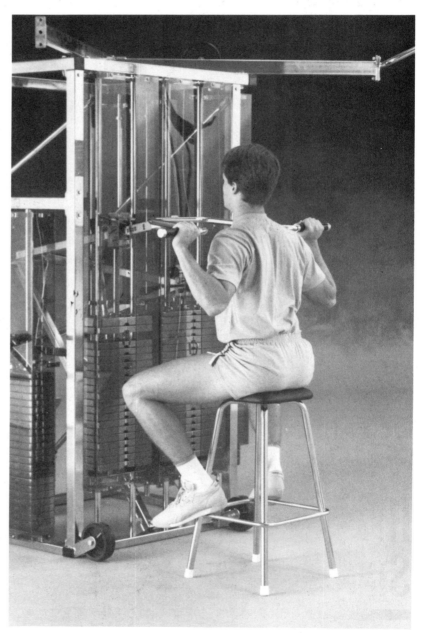

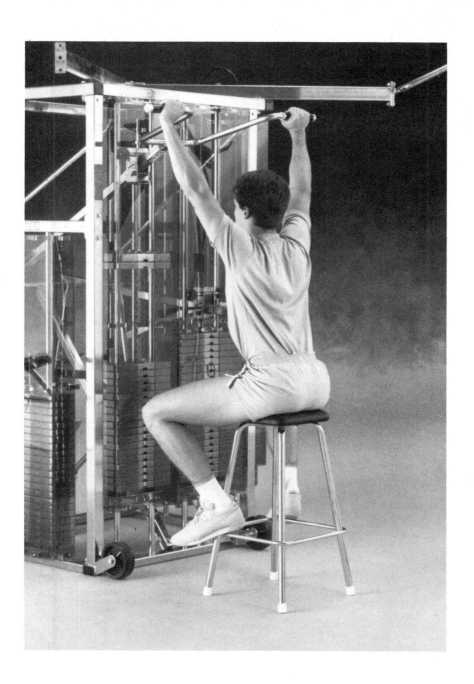

RIGHT- AND LEFT-HAND SINGLE PRESS

To develop your weaker arm, follow the above instructions for the Forward Shoulder Press, but use only one arm at a time.

BACK SHOULDER PRESS

Muscle groups affected:

deltoids, trapezius [upper back], triceps.

Sit facing away from the machine. The handle grips should be in line with the front of your neck. Keep your head level. Exhale as you push the weight up with your hands. Look straight ahead (or down to work the muscles through a longer extension). Extend your arms and hands as high as possible for complete extension. Lower the weight slowly, being careful not to let the weight touch or rest on the stack. Repeat.

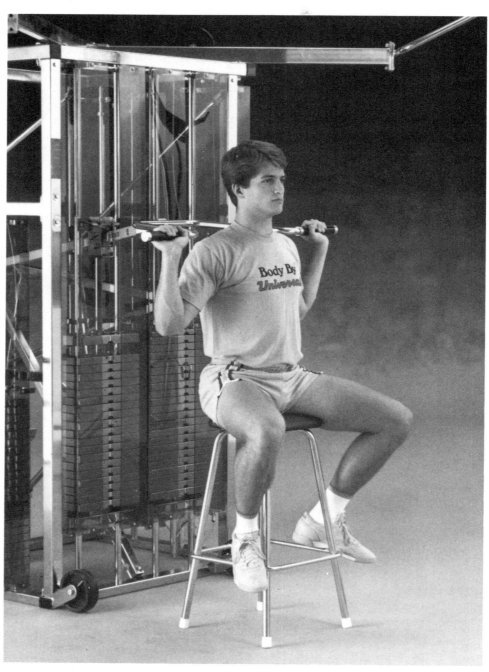

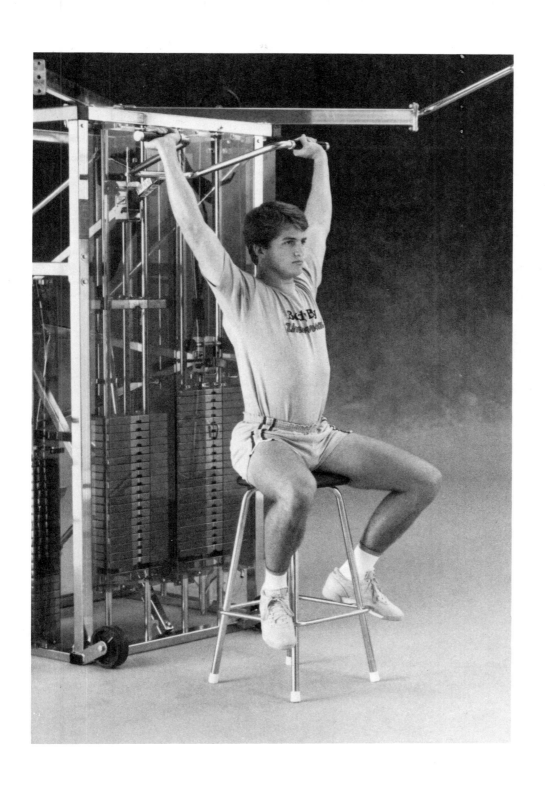

FRENCH CURL (or Triceps Press)

Muscle group affected:

triceps.

Place the stool directly in front of one handle. Sit on the stool, facing away from the machine. Turn and reach back with one hand. Lift the handle up and then grasp it with both hands behind your head. Place your elbows close to your head. Press your hands upward and extend them all the way for the triceps extension. Lower slowly, without letting the weight touch a rest on the stack. Repeat.

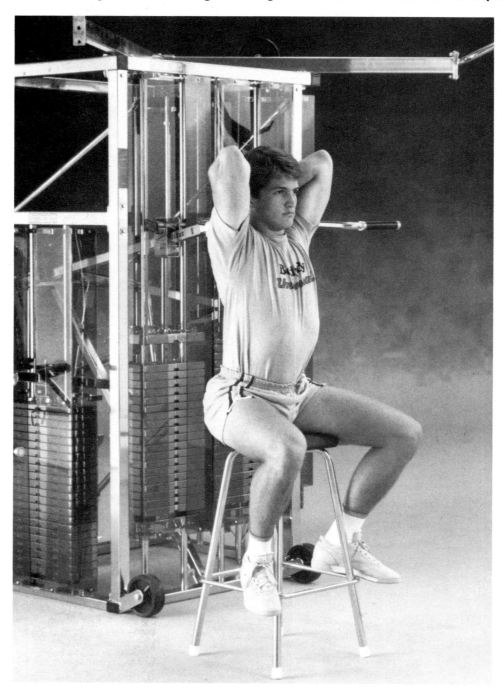

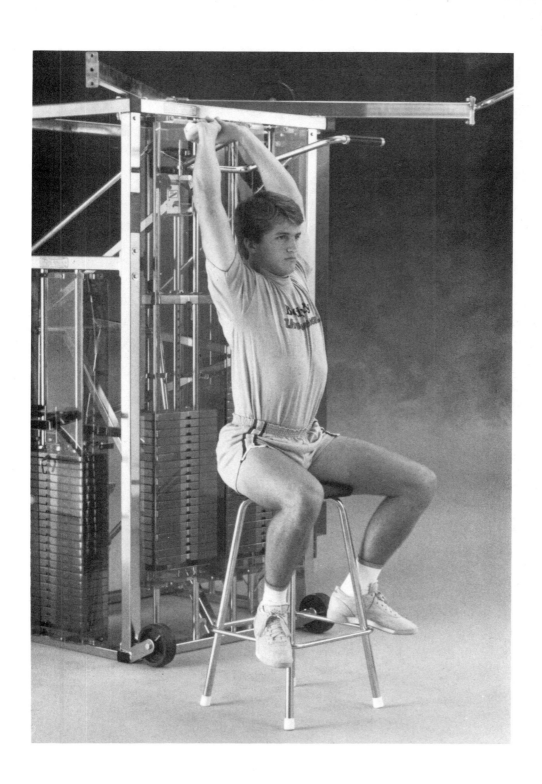

HIGH-LAT EXERCISES

Primary muscle groups affected: latissimus dorsi [back], rhomboids [back], shoulders, biceps, triceps, pectorals [chest].

BACK PULL-DOWN

Kneel facing the machine, directly under the bar. Your back should be straight, your hips in. Using a wide grip, pull the bar down to the back of your neck, exhaling as you do so. Inhale high in your chest and return the weight to its starting position, without letting it rest on the stack. Repeat.

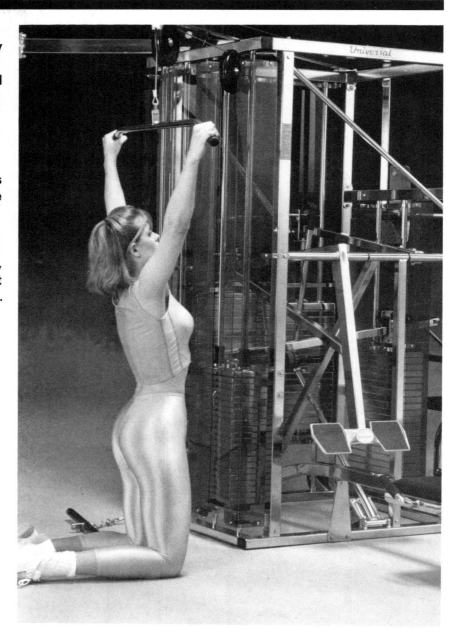

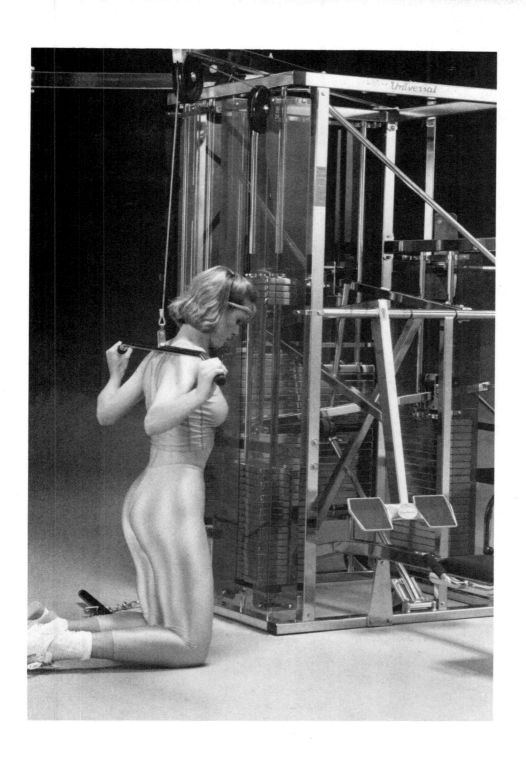

FRONT PULL-DOWN

Muscle groups affected:

the back and the upper arm.

Kneel facing the machine, directly under the bar. Your back should be straight, your hips in. Use a wide grip or a close grip on the bar. Tilt your head back, elevate your chest, and pull the bar to your sternum. Exhale as you bring the weight down; inhale as you return the weight to its starting position without letting the weight touch the remaining stack. If this exercise is too difficult for you, try gripping the bar with one palm toward you, one palm away from you.

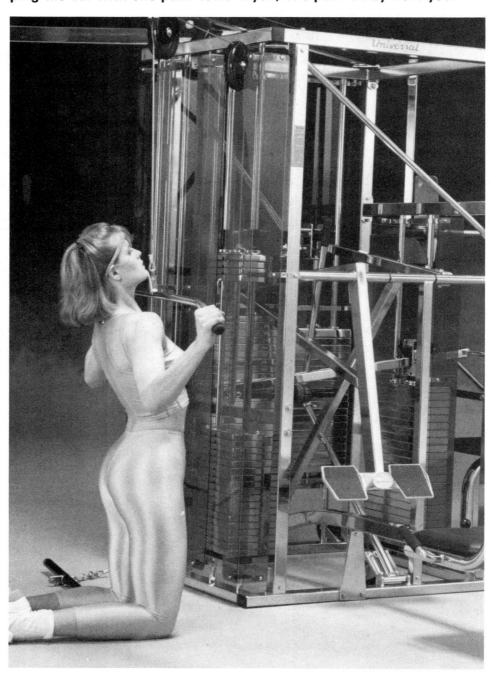

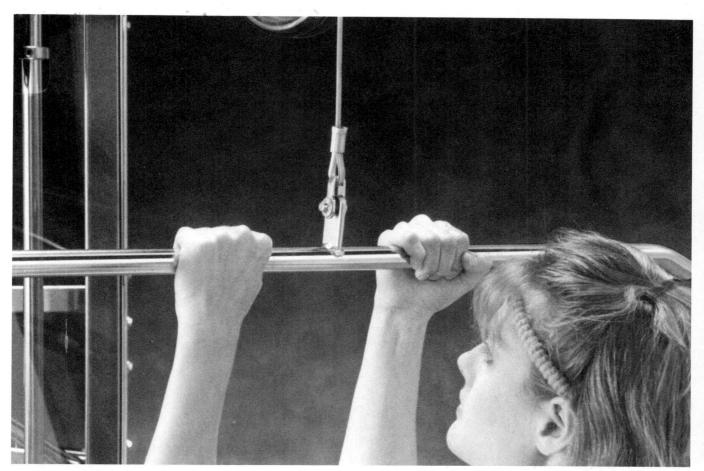

Alternative grip: Front Pull-Down.

HIGH-LAT ABDOMINAL EXERCISE

Muscle groups affected:

abdominals and lower back.

Kneel facing away from the machine. Using a shoulder-width grip, bring the bar to the back of your neck. Keeping the bar at the back of your neck, pull your head toward your knees and your body down. Concentrate on the abdominal pull. Exhale at the bottom of the curl, contracting your abdominal muscles at the same time. Return to the starting position.

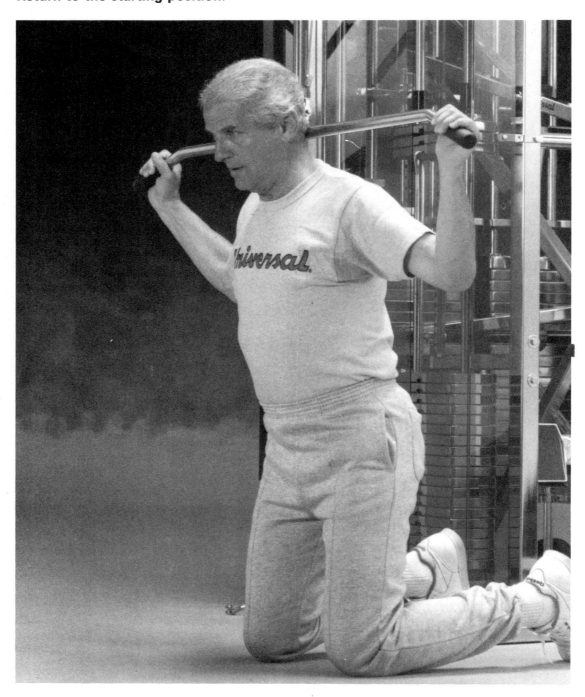

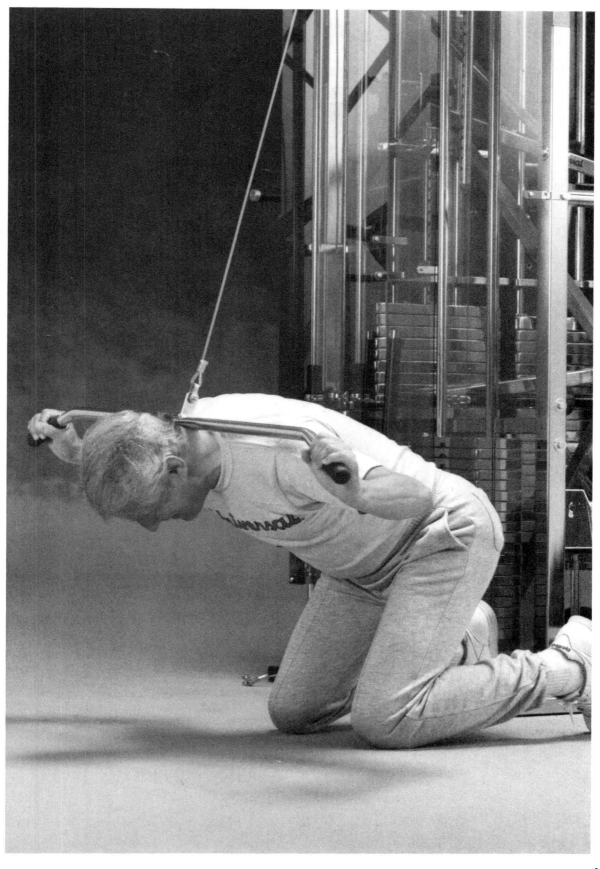

TRICEPS EXTENSION

Standing, grasp the pull-down bar, using a narrow grip. Keeping your elbows at your sides, pull the bar to just below chin height. Flex your triceps as hard as you can as you press the bar down, until your arms are fully extended. Return the weight to its starting position, using control. Exhale as you press the weight down, inhale as you let the weight up. If the cable touches your body, you are using too much weight.

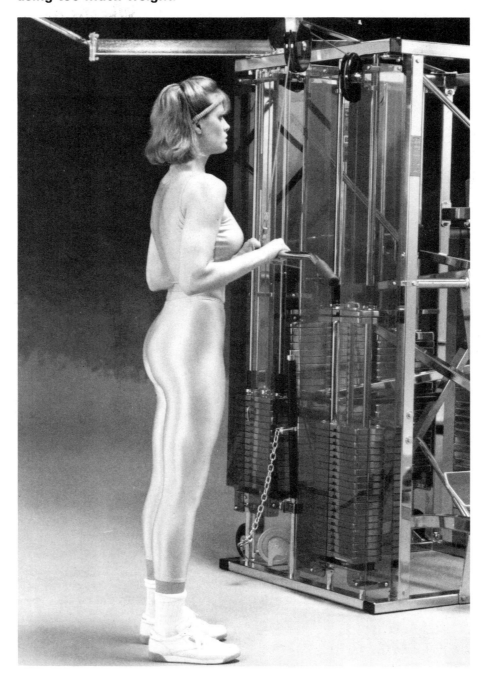

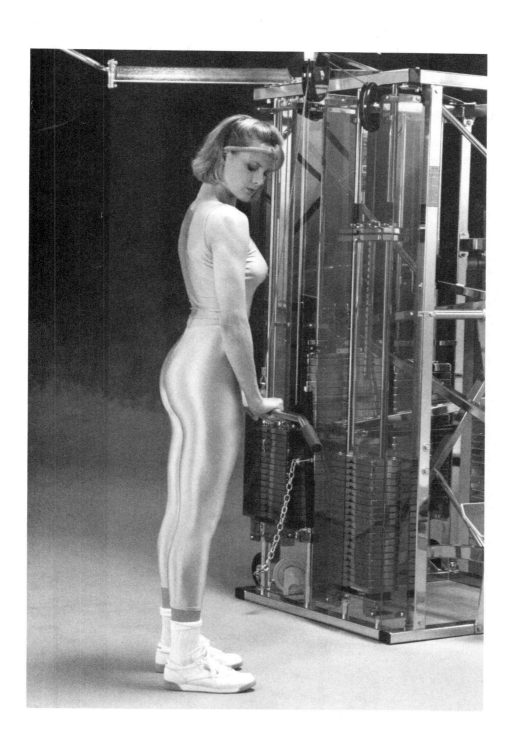

HIGH-LAT ROW

Stand at arm's length from the machine so the cable is stretched tight. Your body should be in an "L" position, with your seat out and your body braced. Using a wide grip, pull the bar to your sternum, exhaling as you bring it down. Extend your arms, inhaling as the weight returns to its starting position. Remember to brace your body to prevent being pulled toward the machine: Keep your body in the "L" position.

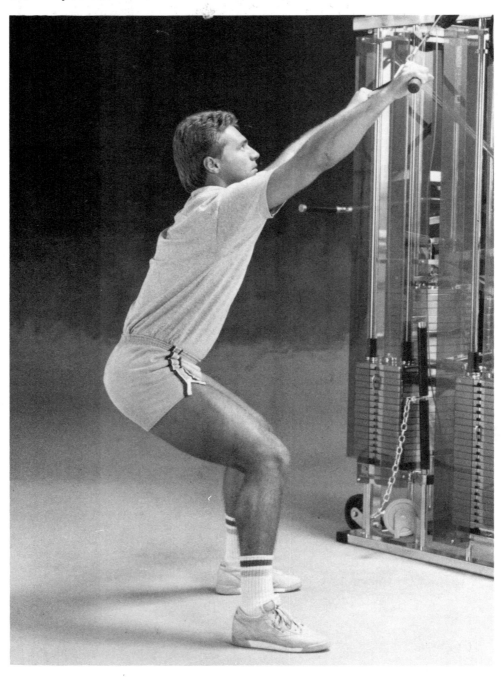

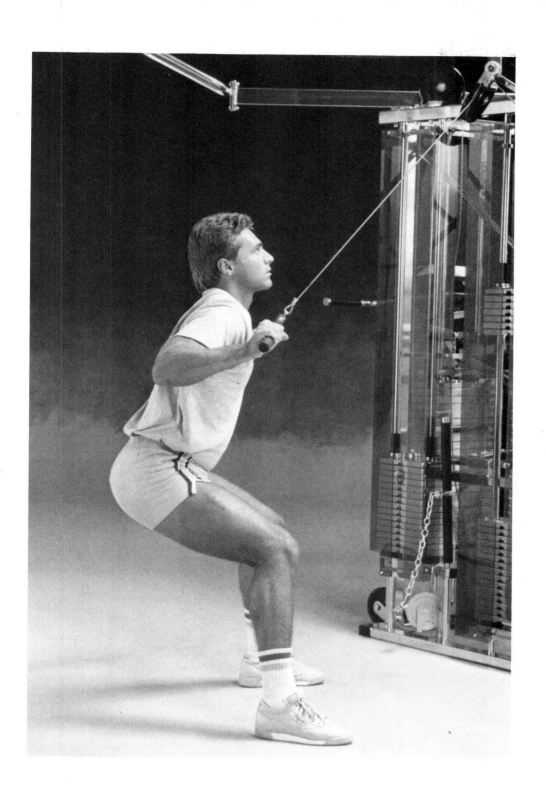

LOW PULLEY STATION EXERCISES

BENT-OVER ROWING (Using Bar or Handles)

Muscle groups affected:

latissimus dorsi [back], rhomboids, trapezius [upper back].

Bend forward at the waist, facing the machine. Grasp the handles shoulder width apart. Keep your back straight, your arms fully extended. Pull the handles to your waist, exhaling as you do so. Inhale while returning handle to starting position. Repeat.

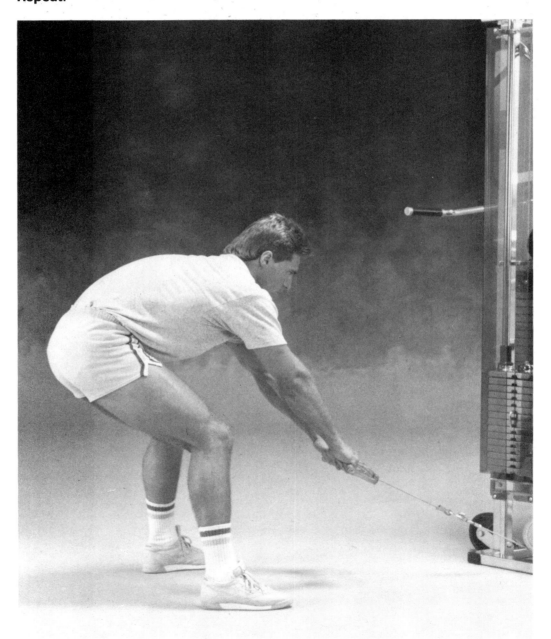

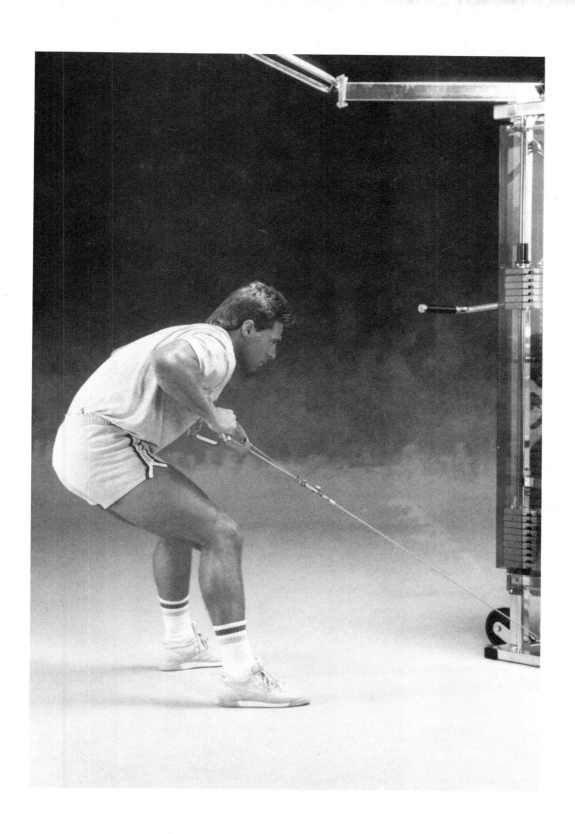

UPRIGHT ROWING

Stand facing the machine. Using a narrow grip, pull your elbows high until your hands are under your chin. Inhale as you bring the weight up; exhale as you slowly lower it back to the starting position. Repeat. If the cable is touching the weight stack, you're standing too close.

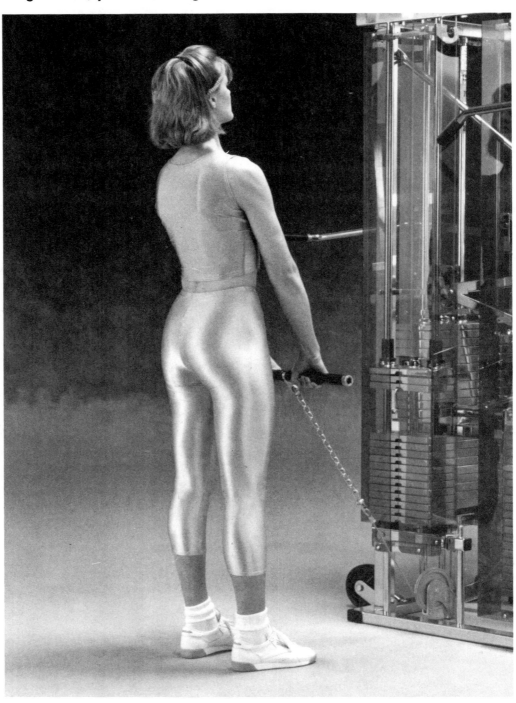

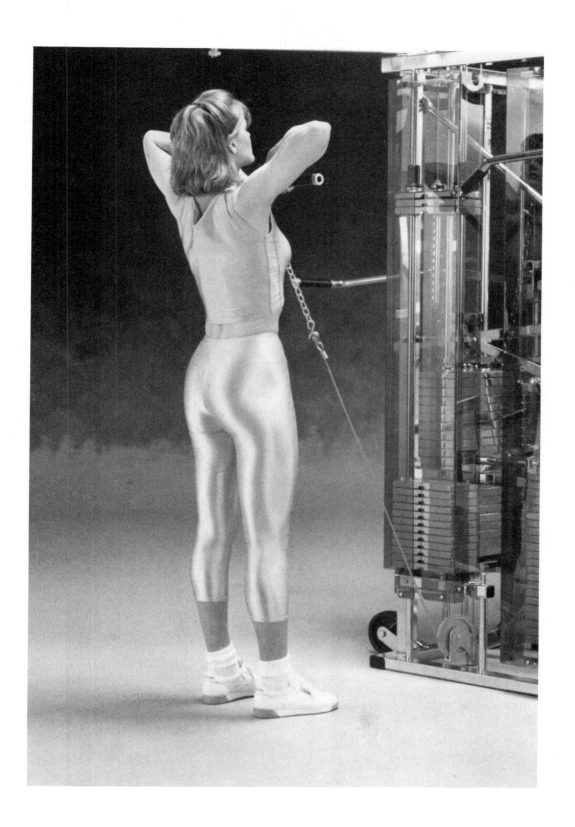

DOUBLE ARM CURL (Using Bar or Handles)

Muscle group affected:

biceps.

Grasp the bar with your palms facing up. Stand with your body braced backward. Bring the bar in an arc to your chest. Inhale as you bring the weight up; exhale as you lower it. Remember to keep your elbows in, and be careful not to arch your back.

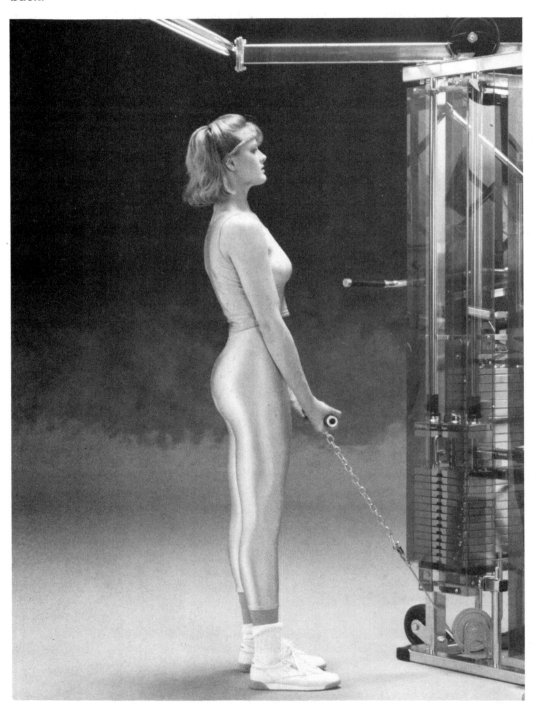

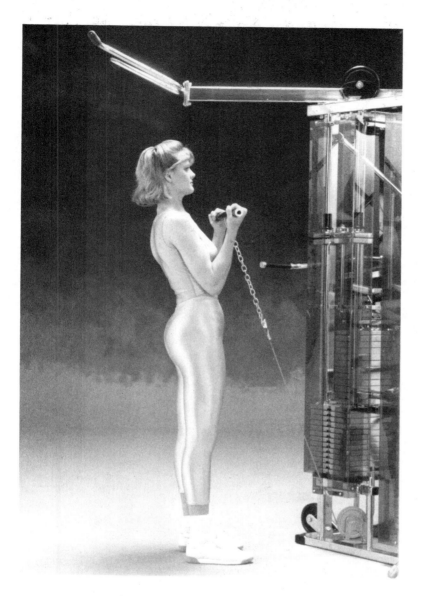

REVERSE ARM CURL

Follow the instructions for the Double Arm Curl, but with your palms facing down.

ALTERNATE ARM CURL
(Using Stirrup Handles)

Bend one arm and bring it to your shoulder. As that arm returns to its starting position, bend your other arm and bring it to your shoulder.

RIP-UP (Using Bar or Handles)

Muscle groups affected:

trapezius [upper back], deltoids, rhomboids.

Facing away from the machine, bend over and grasp the bar through your legs, using a narrow grip. Pull your hands up through your legs until the bar is close to your body under your chin. To help bring the bar through your legs, and reduce strain on your back, step forward with your right or left foot, using short steps.

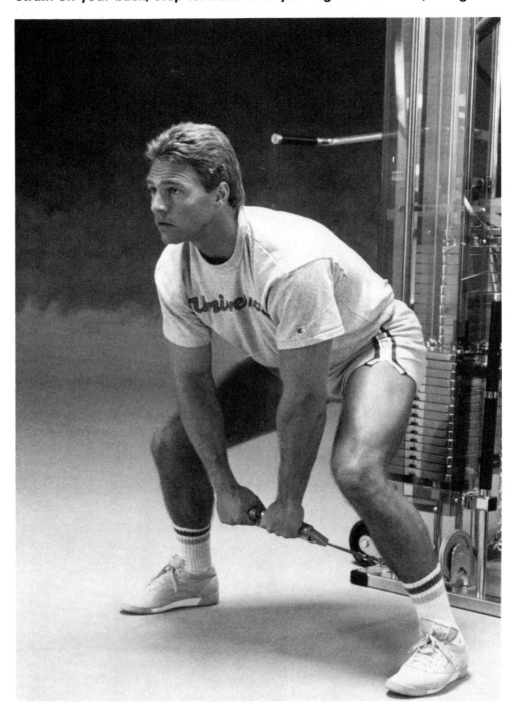

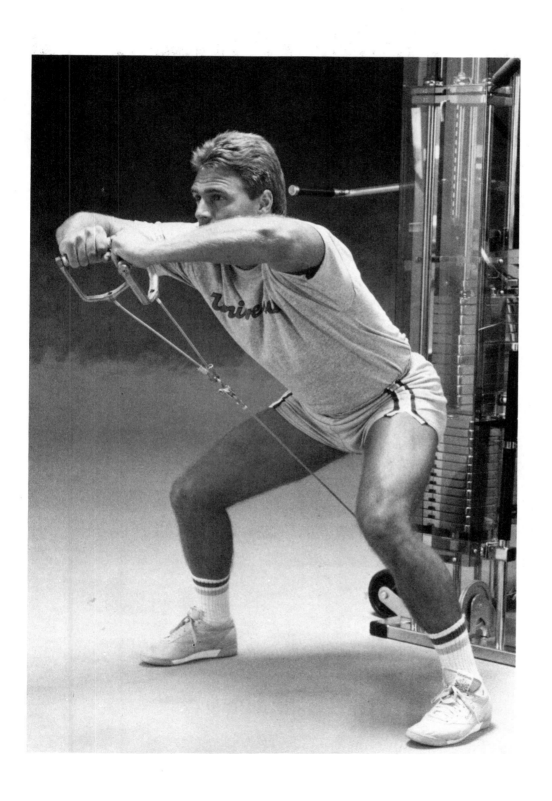

PULL-OVER (Using Bar or Handles)

Muscle groups affected:

latissimus dorsi [back], pectorals, rib muscles.

Lie on your back with your legs extended and your head toward the machine. Place your arms straight over your head and grasp the bar using a shoulder-width grip. Pull the bar in an arc to your waist. Exhale at the end of the pull. Inhale while you return your arms to the starting position. Repeat.

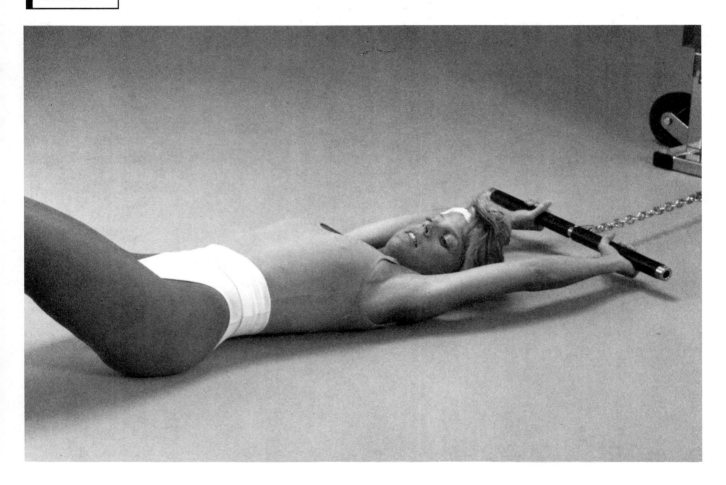

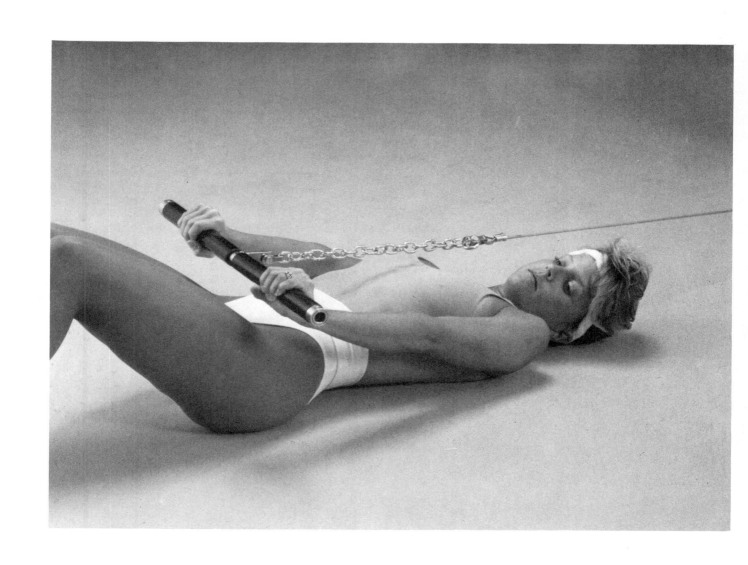

BENT ARM PULL-OVER
(Using Bar or Handles)

Lie on the floor. Bend your arms at a ninety-degree angle. Extend your arms behind and below your head, keeping your elbows up close to your head. Grasp the bar and pull it to your sternum, exhaling at the end of the pull. Inhale while returning your arms to the starting position. Repeat.

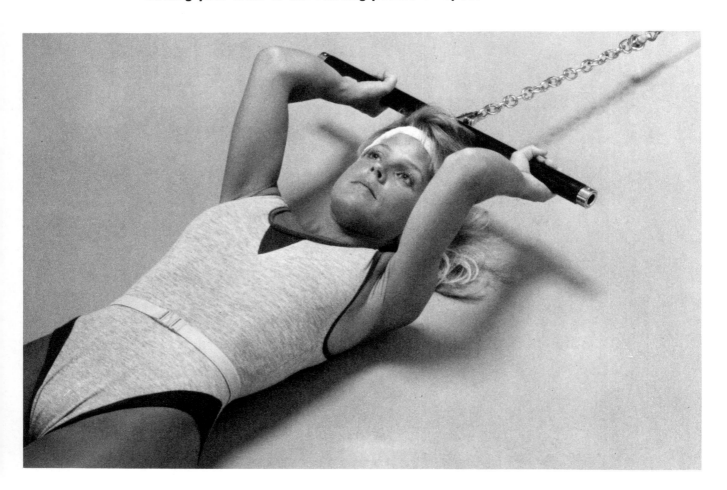

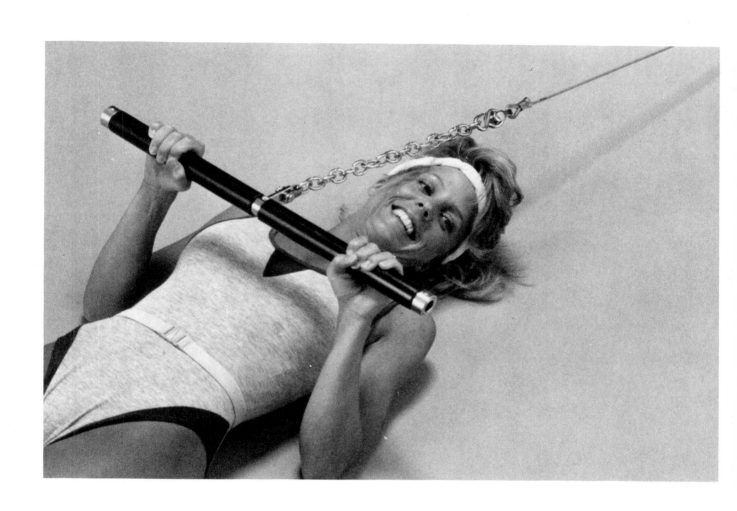

FRONT RAISE (Using Bar or Handles)

Muscle groups affected:

deltoids, trapezius [upper back].

Lie on your back with your feet facing the machine. Reach down and pull the bar through a complete arc (keep your arms locked) until your arms extend over your head. Inhale as you bring the weight up; exhale on the return, breathing high in your chest. Repeat.

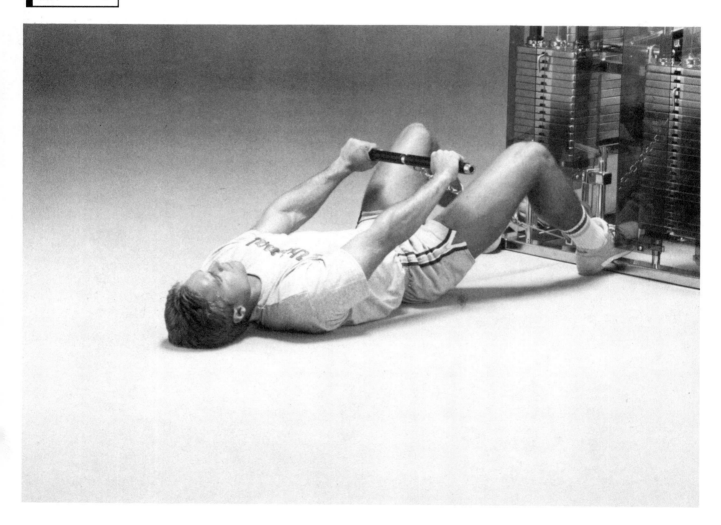

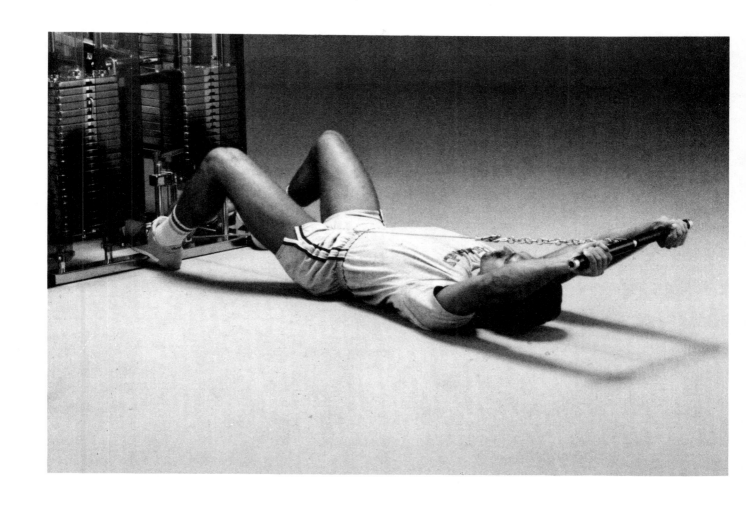

ALTERNATE FRONT RAISE

Repeat the instructions above, using one arm at a time.

LATERAL RAISE (Using Bar or Handles)

Muscle groups affected:

pectorals, deltoids.

Lie on your back on the floor, parallel to the machine, with your right arm extended across your body. Pull the handle across the center of your body. Exhale at the conclusion of the pull. Reverse your position and do the exercise using your other arm.

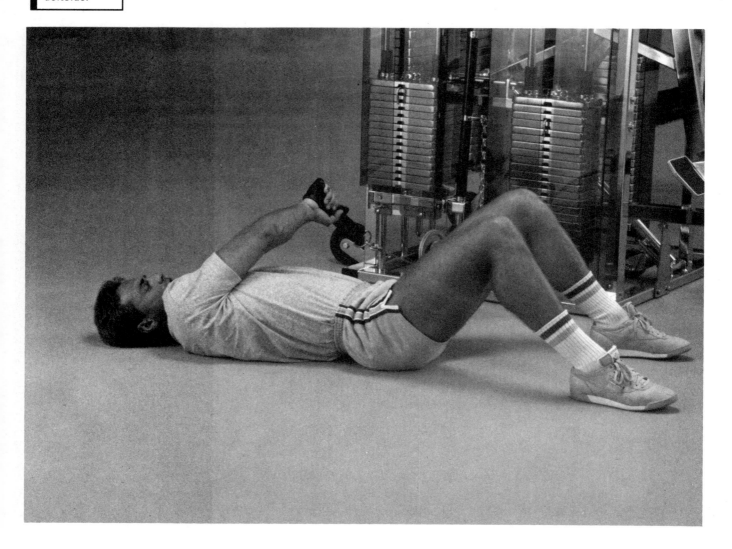

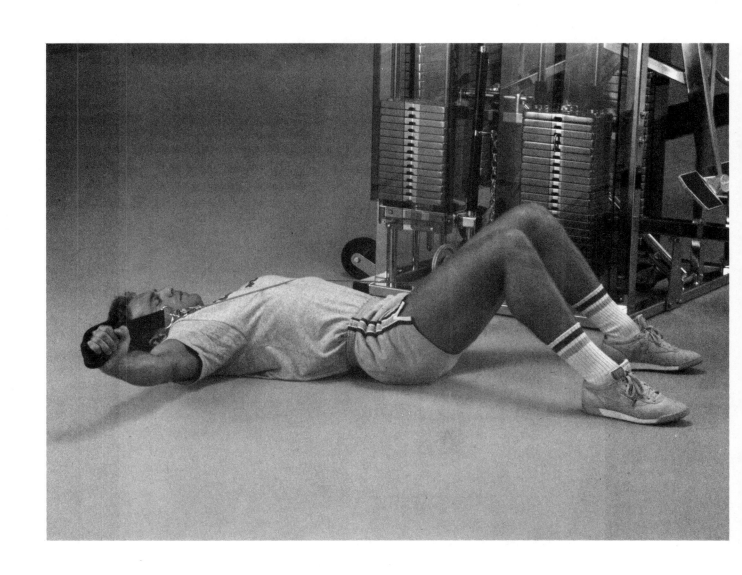

SIDE BEND (Using Bar or Handles)

Stand with your side to the machine, with your feet shoulder-width apart. Grasp the bar with your near hand and pull up. Your arm should hang straight and fully extended. Bend your free arm and place it behind your legs. Bend to the outside as far as possible, controlling the weight up and down.

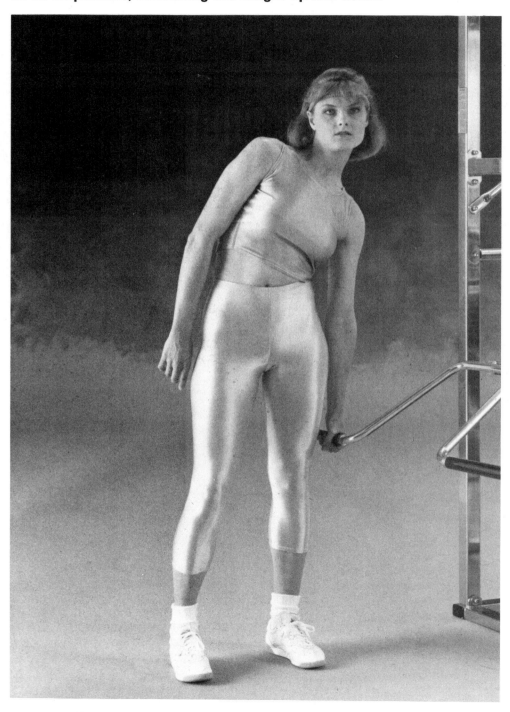

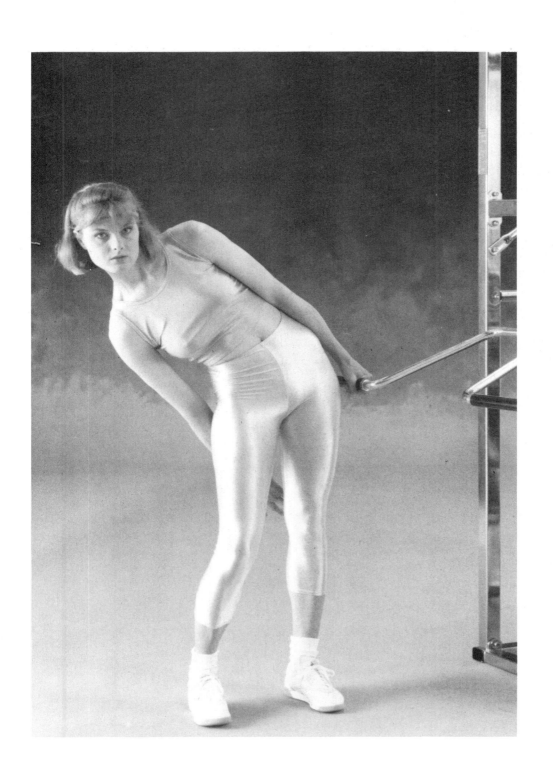

WRIST CURL (Using Bar or Handles)

Kneel facing the machine. Grasp the bar with your palm facing up, your forearm resting on your knee. Using only your wrist, curl the bar toward your body. Repeat.

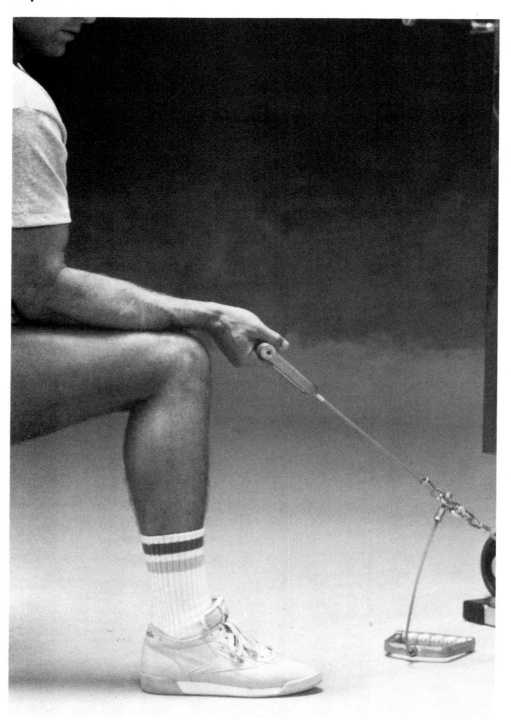

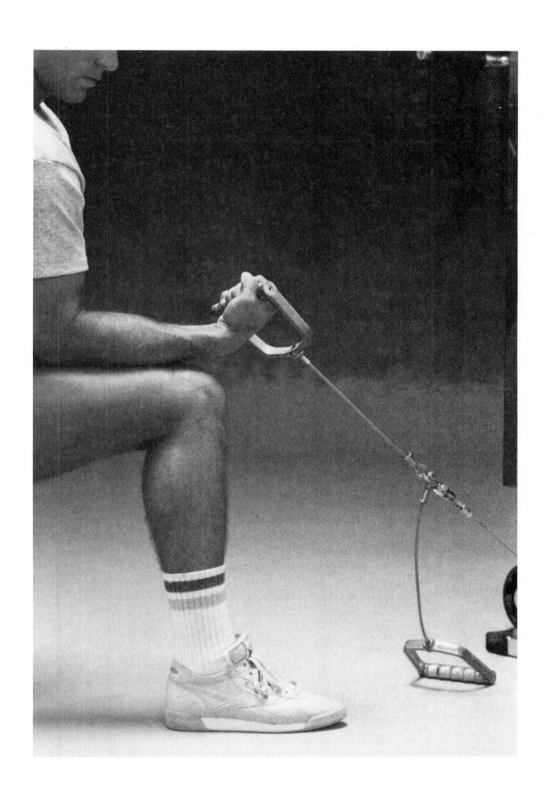

REVERSE WRIST CURL (Using Bar or Handles)

Muscle groups affected:

extensors of wrist, hand, and forearm.

Kneel facing the machine. Grasp the bar with your palm down, your forearm resting on your bent leg. Pull the back of your hand toward your forearm, using only the wrist. Repeat.

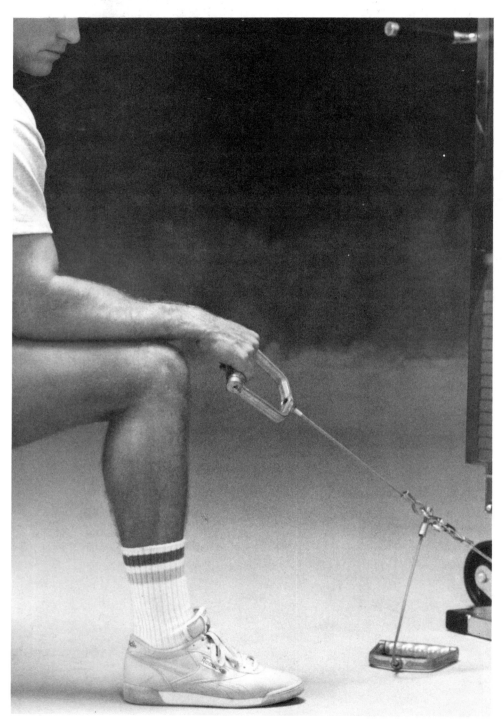

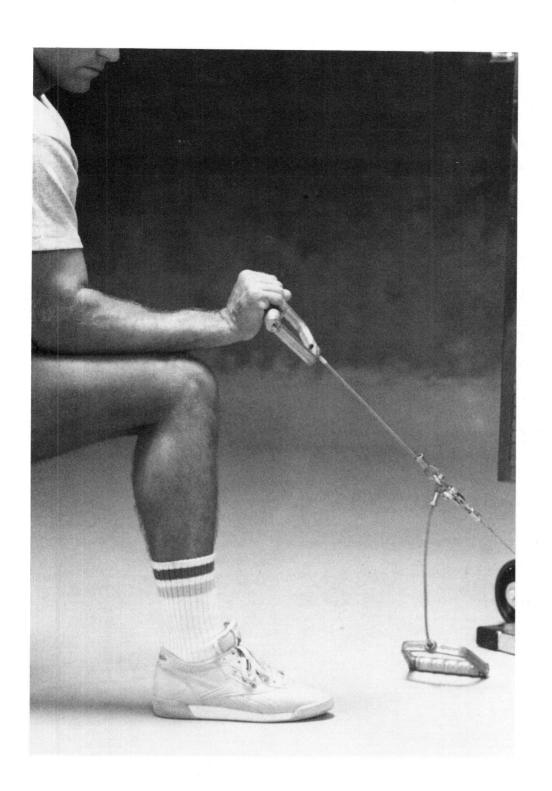

DEAD LIFT AND SHOULDER SHRUG (Using Bar or Handles) (Advanced Exercise)

Muscle groups affected:

upper and lower back.

Facing the machine, bend at the waist, keeping your back straight and your head up. Grasp the bar using a shoulder-width grip. You should be far enough back so that your arms are straight. Brace your feet and pull the bar until you straighten up past an upright position. Pull your shoulders up and roll them back. Inhale high in your chest while bringing the bar forward. Exhale while bending forward by contracting the abdominal muscles.

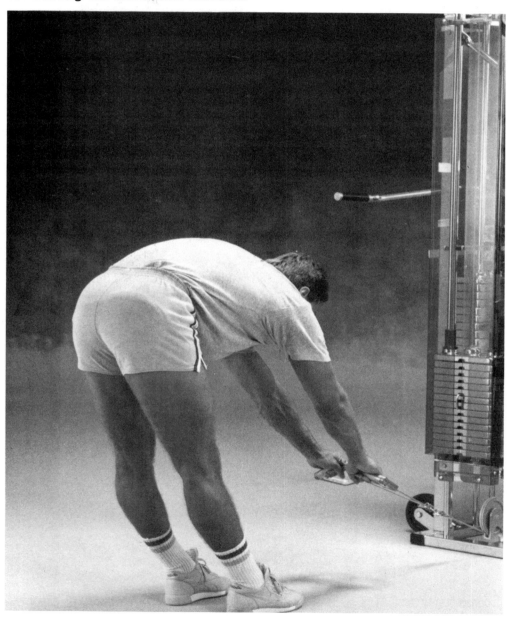

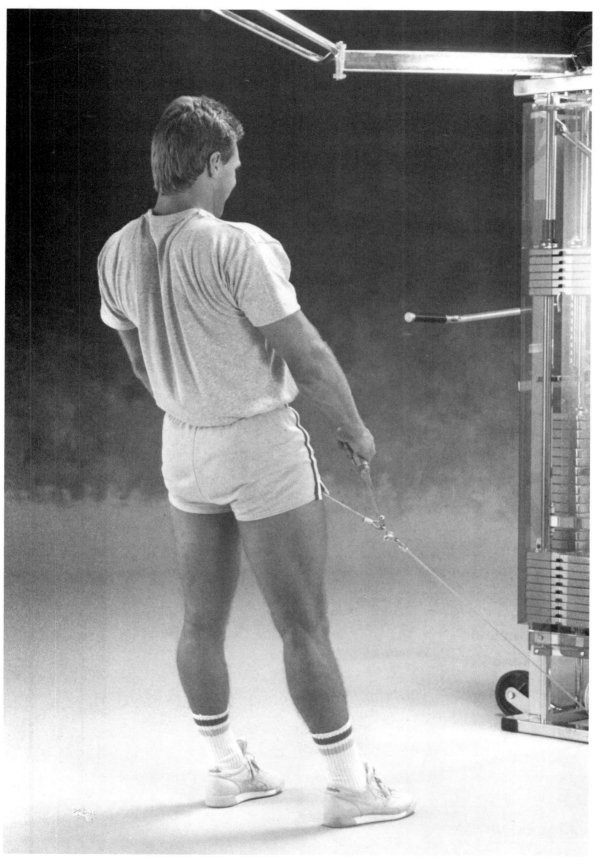

CHINNING EXERCISES

Primary muscle groups affected: biceps, latissimus dorsi [back], trapezius [upper back], shoulder, deltoids [shoulder], triceps, forearm.

REVERSE GRIP CHIN

This exercise is very difficult because of the radial forearm muscles involved. Grab the handles using a reverse grip (palms facing away from you). To prevent yourself from cheating by kicking your legs, cross them and bend your knees. From a hanging position, pull yourself up until your chin is above the level of the handles. Control your body on the way down. Repeat.

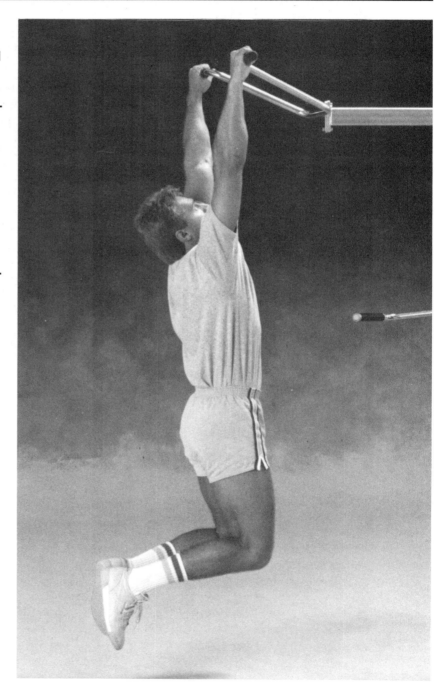

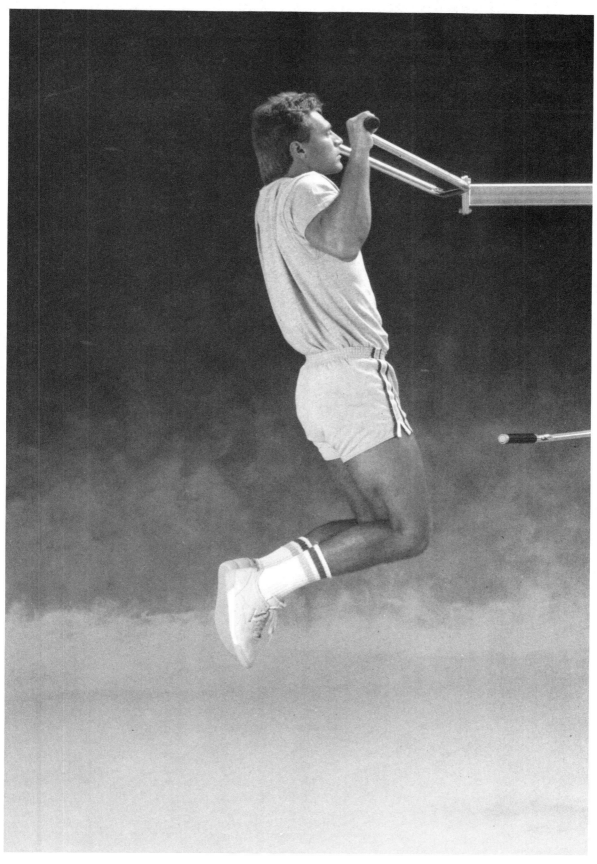

REGULAR GRIP CHIN

This exercise is less difficult than the reverse grip chin because you can use your forearms to help pull yourself up. Grab the handles using a regular grip (palms facing toward you). To prevent yourself from cheating by kicking your legs, cross them and bend your knees. From a hanging position, pull yourself up until your chin is above the level of the handles. Control any body swing on the way down. Repeat.

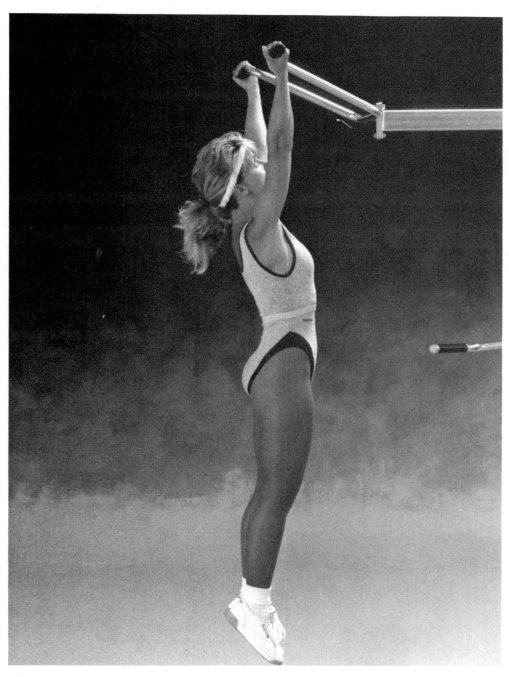

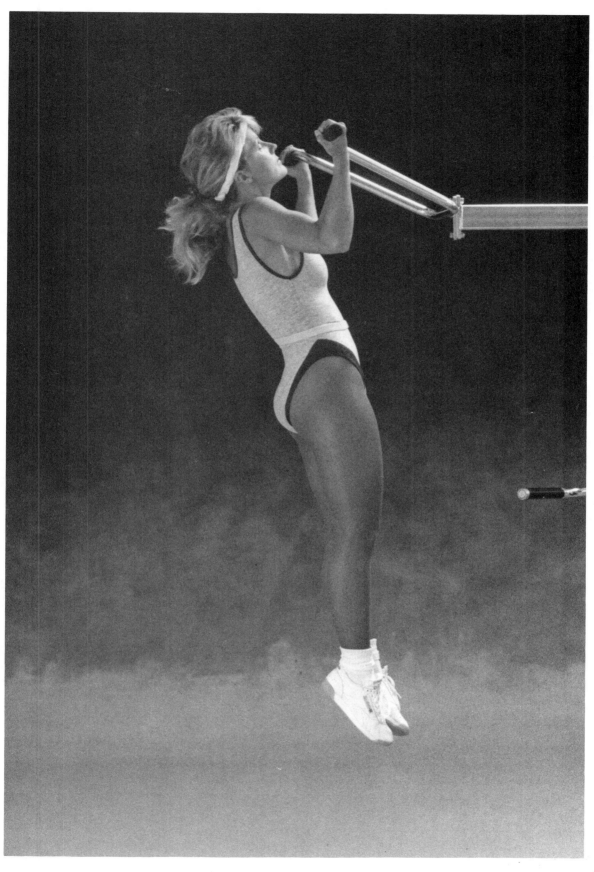

SHOULDER BROADENER

Another tough exercise. Grab the handles using a wide reverse grip. From a hanging position, pull your shoulders straight up, keeping your head down and forward.

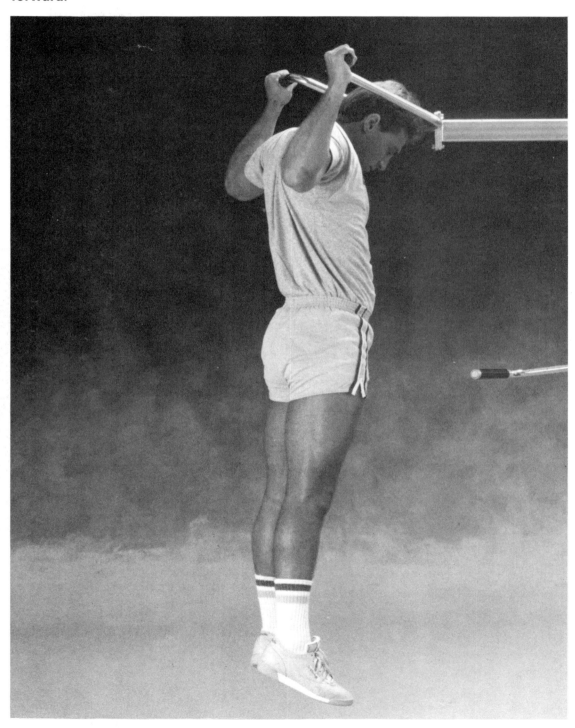

DIPPING EXERCISES

Primary muscle groups affected: trapezius [upper back], latissimus dorsi [back], deltoids [shoulder], triceps.

DIP

Facing the machine, grasp the handles. Hoist yourself to an upright position on the bars, keeping your arms straight and your elbows locked. Bend your knees (if you have a tendency to swing your legs, cross your feet to prevent this). Bending your arms at the elbows, lower yourself until your upper arms are parallel to the floor, inhaling as you descend. Push yourself back up to the starting position, exhaling as you ascend.

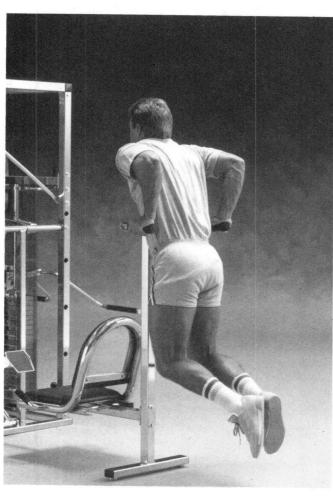
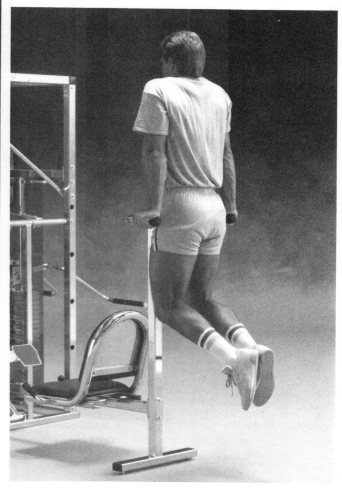

REVERSE GRIP DIP

This exercise is much more difficult than regular dips, because it relies almost exclusively on the strength of your triceps muscles. Facing the machine, grasp the handles with your hands facing in. Hoist yourself to an upright position on the bars, keeping your arms straight and your elbows locked. Cross your feet and bend your knees. Bending your arms at the elbows, lower yourself to the bar, inhaling as you descend, until your upper arms are parallel to the floor. Push yourself back up to the starting position, exhaling as you ascend.

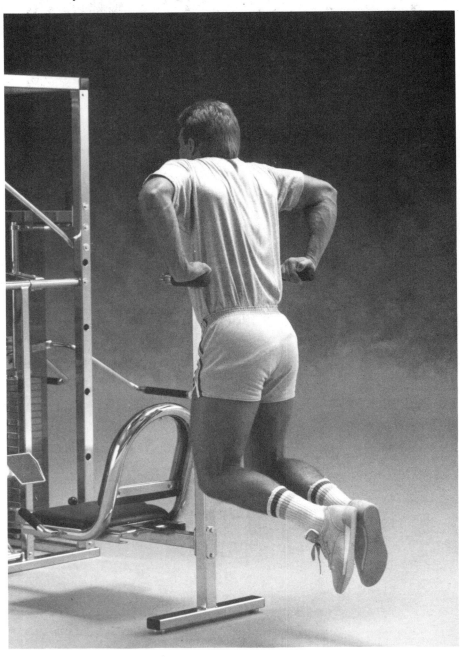

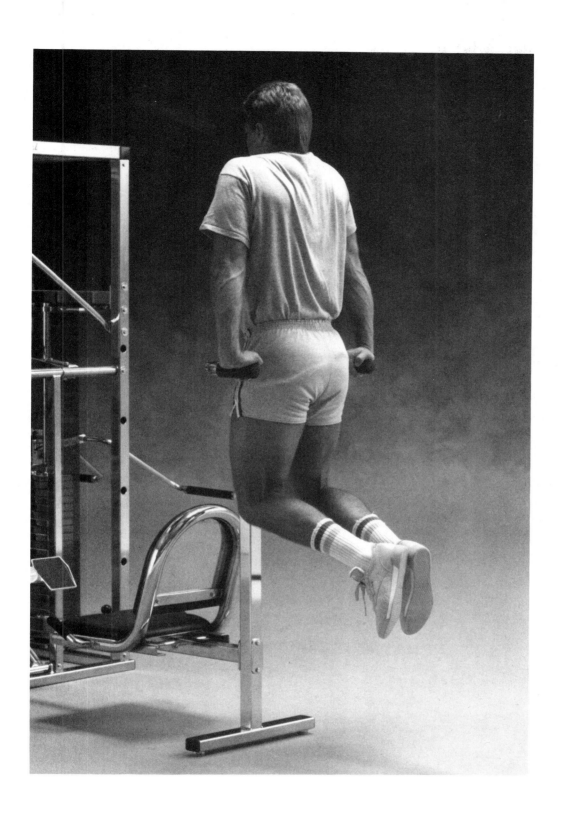

SEATED PULL-UP WITHOUT BENCH

Sit on the floor, facing away from the machine, with your legs out straight. Grasp the handles with your palms facing in. Pull up with your arms until your shoulders touch your hands, then straighten your body. Emphasize pulling your chest up. Exhale as you pull up, inhale as you return to the starting position. To make the exercise more difficult, you can place your heels on a bench in front of you. (Note: this is a beginning exercise for those who are unable to perform a chin-up.)

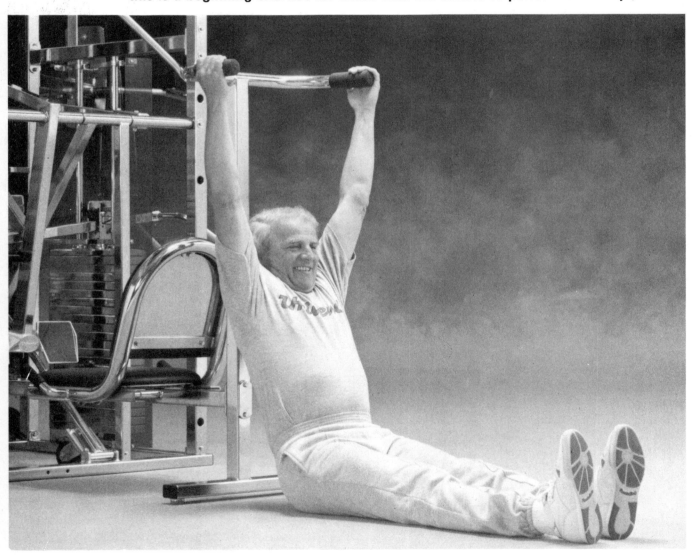

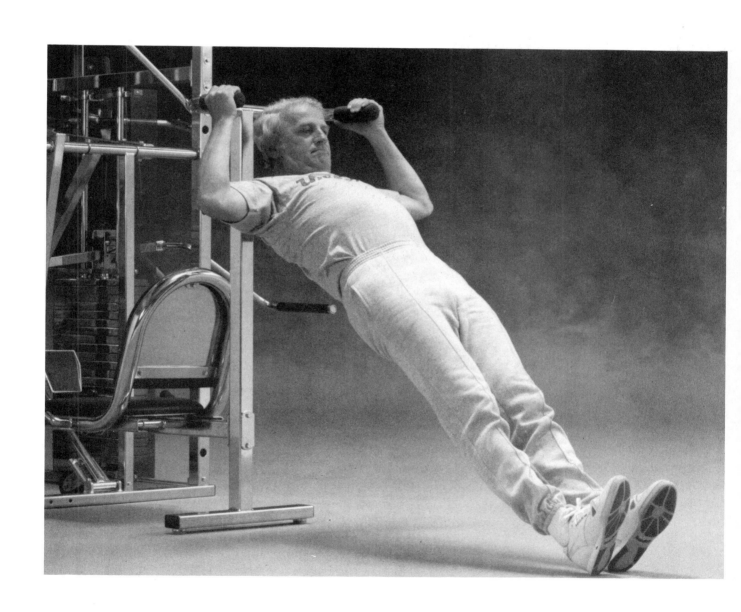

NECK CONDITIONING STATION EXERCISE

BACKWARD NECK EXTENSION
(Using Head Harness)

Muscle groups affected:

all neck muscles.

Place the head harness around your head. Facing the machine, brace one arm on the machine or the handle and pull your head backward as far as possible. Slowly, return to the starting position and repeat. Use *moderate* resistance.

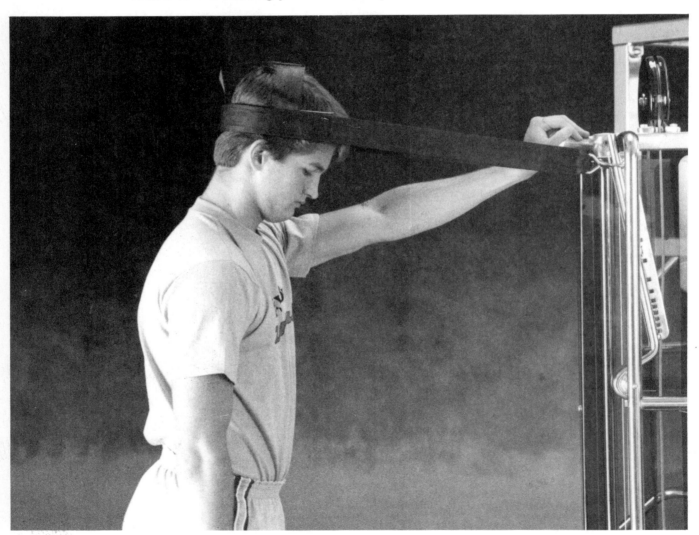

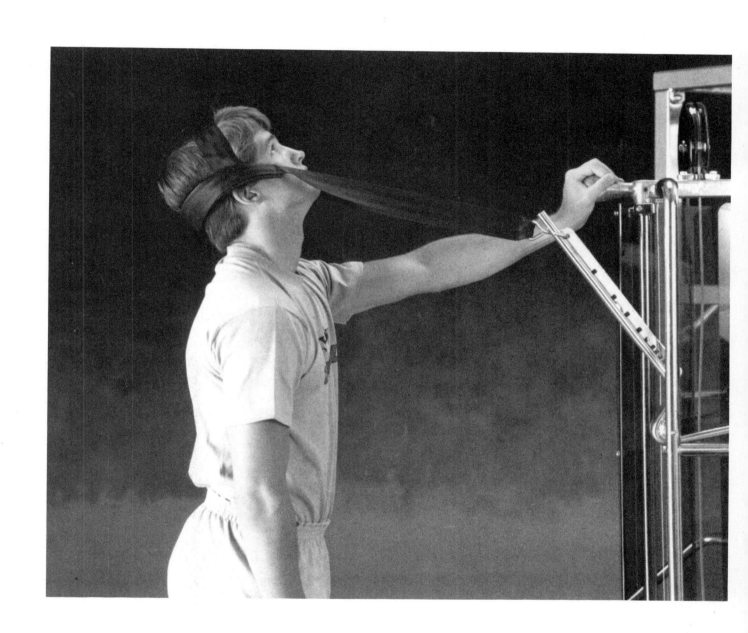

RIGHT SIDE NECK EXTENSION
(Using Head Harness)

Stand parallel to the machine, left side in, and place the harness on your head sideways. Pull your head toward your right shoulder, controlling the motion carefully.

LEFT SIDE NECK EXTENSION
(Using Head Harness)

Stand parallel to the machine, right side in, and place the harness on your head sideways. Pull your head toward your left shoulder, controlling the motion carefully.

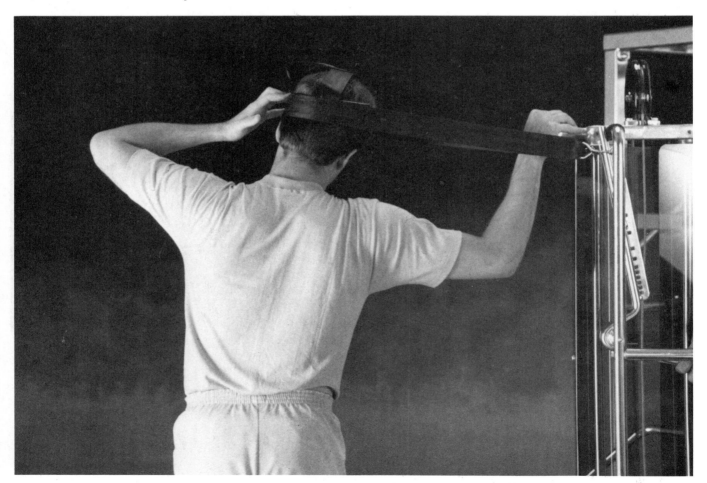

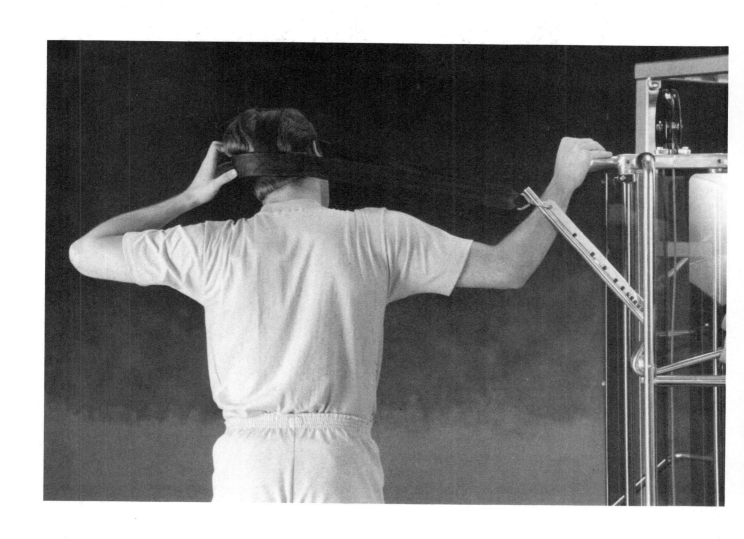

Forward Neck Extension

Facing away from the machine, place the head harness on your head. Brace your body by placing your hands on your knees. Extend your chin forward and down toward your chest. Slowly and with control, return your head to the starting position. Repeat the exercise.

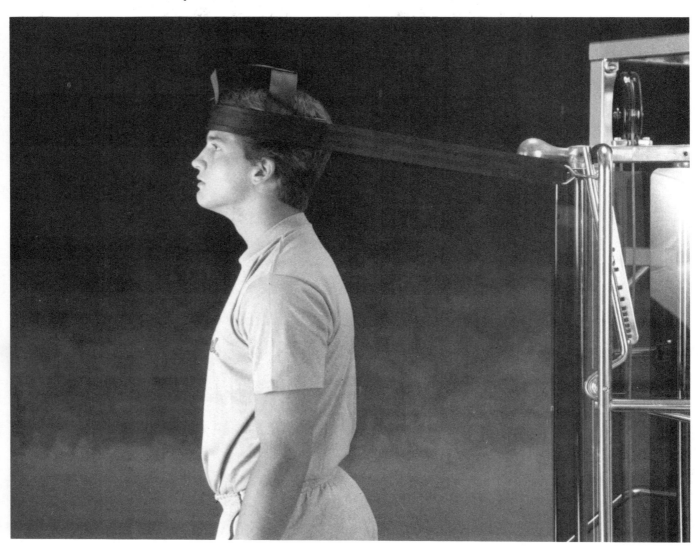

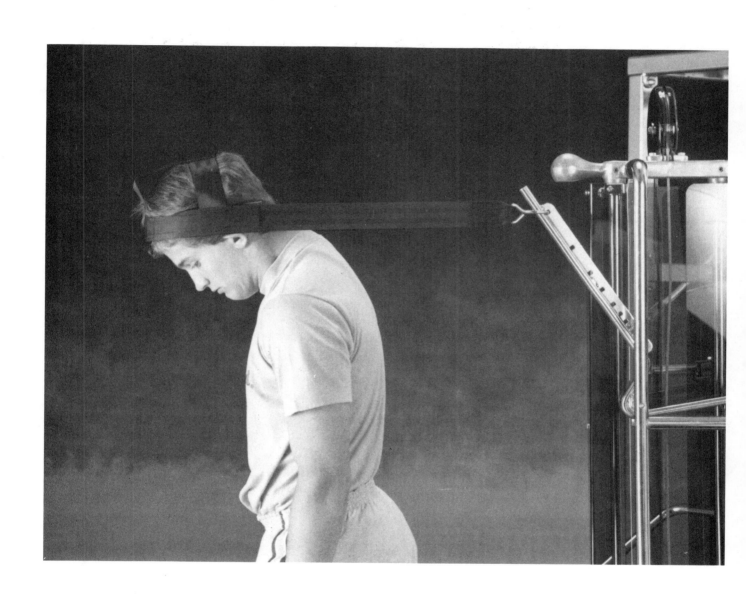

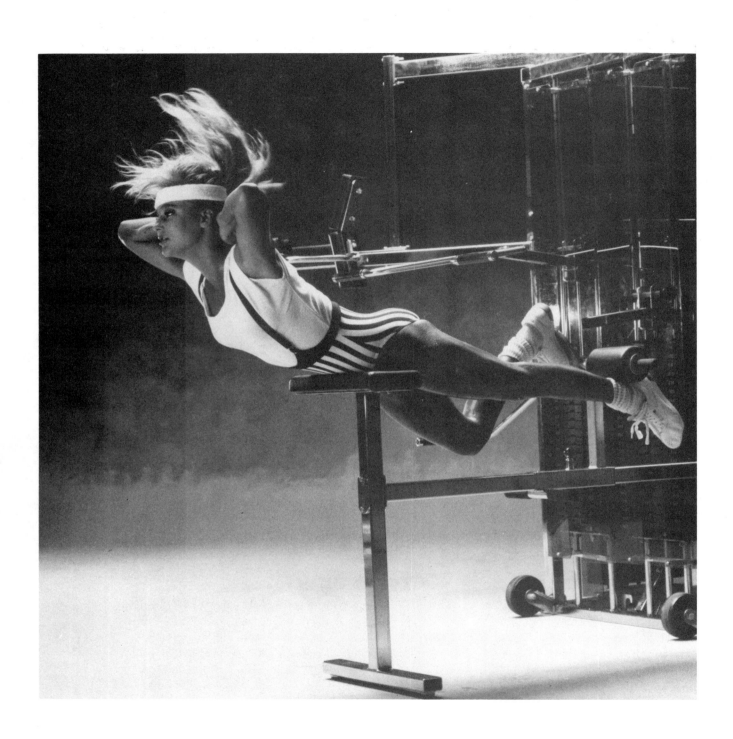

8

TRAINING AND BUILDING THE ABDOMINALS AND LOWER BACK

Perhaps the most overlooked area of the body in terms of general fitness is the abdominals and lower back. Because so many of us lead a sedentary lifestyle— most of us spent 95% of our waking hours in a seated position—over 80% of all Americans suffer from weak lower back muscles. This is a major cause of back pain later in life. With our sedentary lifestyle, developing and maintaining a strong lower back and strong abdominal muscles is more important than ever. You need a good solid base for the rest of the body—and only a strong torso can give you that. Developing this part of your body will also help prevent injury.

HIP FLEXOR EXERCISES/ CHINNING STATION

Muscle groups affected: hip flexors, rib muscles, lower abdominals.

HIP FLEXOR

Facing away from the machine, place your elbows on the pads and grasp the handles. Pull your knees to your chest, maintaining control as you bring your legs up and down. Exhale as your knees come to your chest, inhale as your legs return to the starting position.

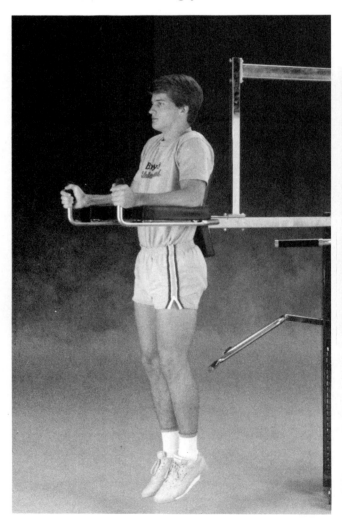

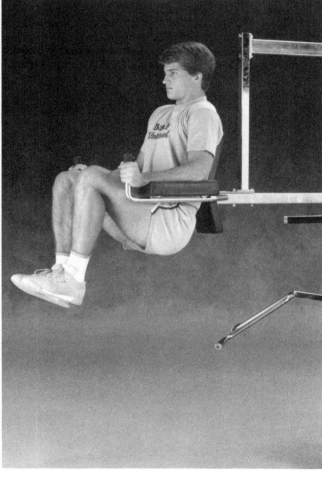

ALTERNATE HIP FLEXOR

Follow the instructions for the hip flexor exercise, but alternate raising your legs.

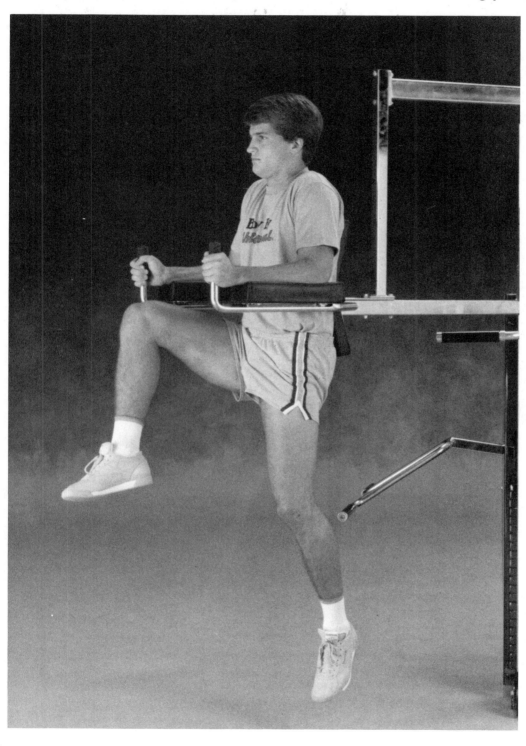

DOUBLE STRAIGHT LEG RAISE

Facing away from the machine, place your elbows on the pads and grasp the handles. Without bending your knees, lift both legs until they extend parallel to the floor. Lower your legs slowly and repeat.

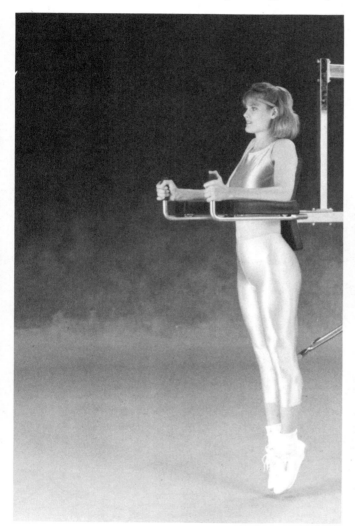

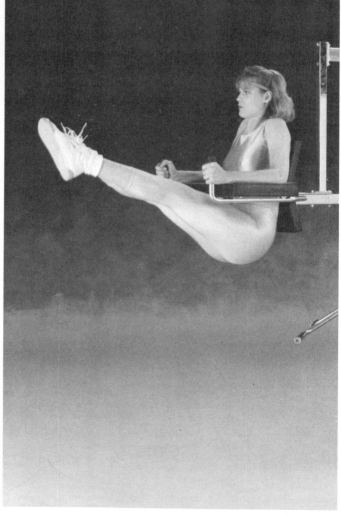

ALTERNATE STRAIGHT LEG RAISE

Follow the instructions for leg raises, but raise each leg alternately.

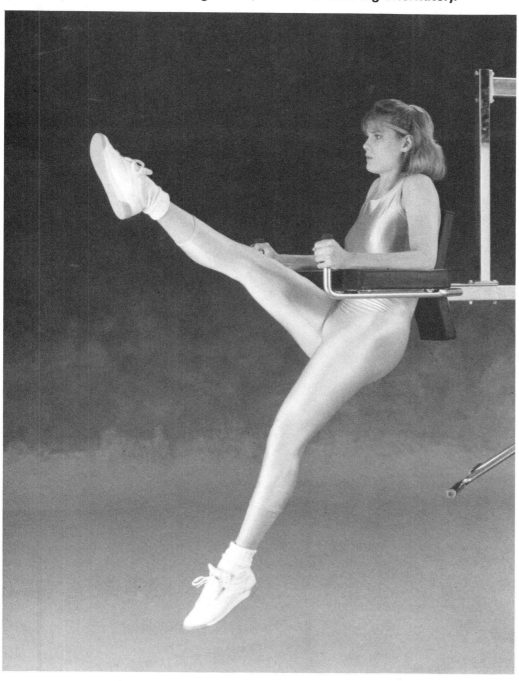

ABDOMINAL BOARD EXERCISES

General instructions: The height adjustment on the board depends on your strength and ability. It's important that beginners do not overdo it. Start with board at its lowest position.

Primary muscle groups affected: upper internal and external obliques, hip flexors, quadriceps.

CRUNCH SIT-UP

Lying on your back, hook your feet under the rollers, bending your knees. Three arm-hand positions are possible for varying the level of difficulty: overhead (easiest), crossed arms in front of your chest (medium difficulty), hands behind head (most difficult). Curl your chin toward your knees, forcefully contracting your abdominal muscles. Don't go all the way up. Exhale on the way up, inhale on the way down.

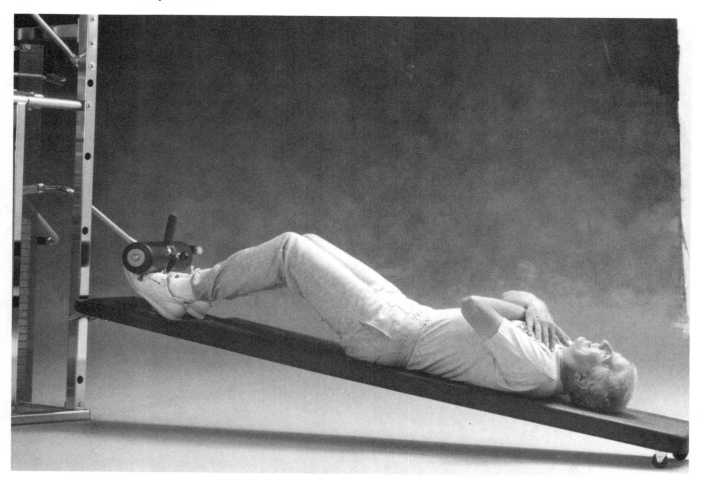

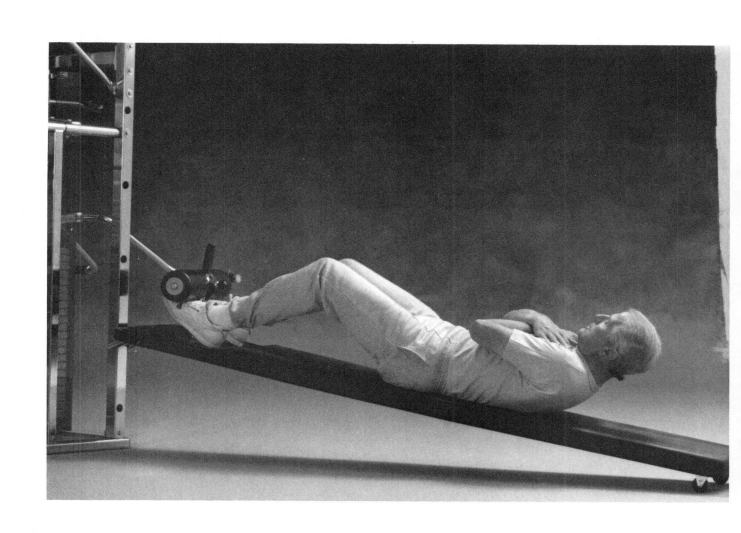

BENT-KNEE TWISTING SIT-UP

Position your body as described in the Crunch Sit-Up, but at the top of the sit-up curl, twist so your right elbow touches your left knee. On the next curl, twist so your left elbow touches your right knee. The extra twist increases the difficulty and works the external oblique muscles.

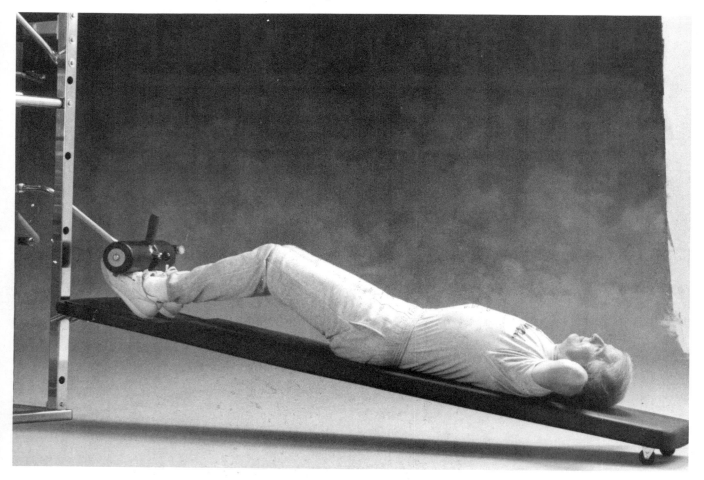

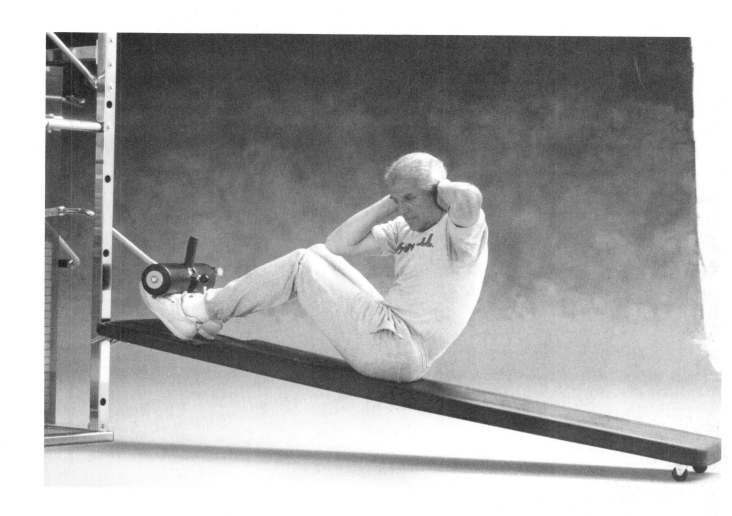

Bent-Knee Double Twisting Sit-Up

Position your body as described in the Crunch Sit-Up, with your hands behind your head, fingers interlaced. Sit up. At the top of the sit-up, twist your left elbow to your right knee and then your right elbow to your left knee. Return to center, then return to the starting position. This is the most difficult type of sit-up.

ALTERNATE BENT-KNEE LEG RAISE

Lying on your back with your head toward the rollers, grasp the handle with both hands, keeping your shoulders flat. Pull one knee to your chest. Exhale and contract your abdominals when your knee reaches your chest. With your toes pointed, lower your foot and repeat the exercise with your other leg.

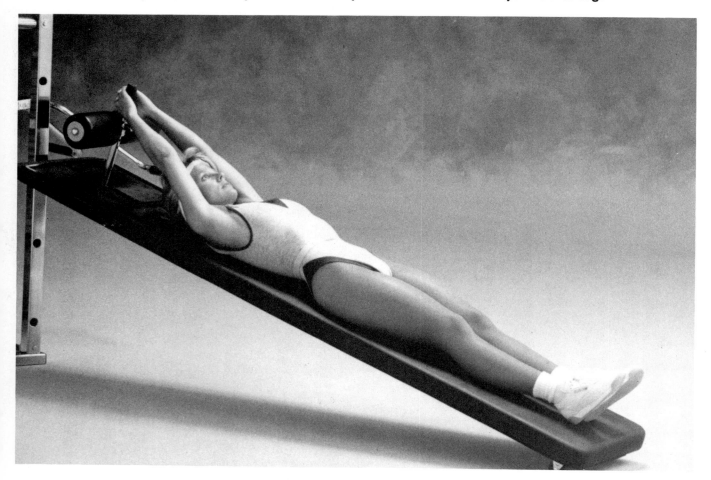

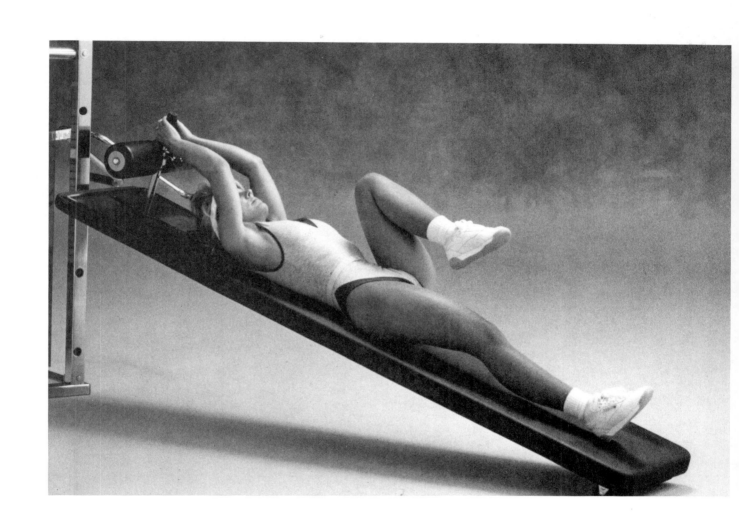

DOUBLE BENT-KNEE LEG RAISE

Lying on your back with your head toward the rollers, grasp the handle with both hands, keeping your shoulders flat. Roll your hips up to raise—and take stress off—your lower back. Pull both knees to your chest. Exhale and contract your abdominals when your knees reach your chest. With your toes pointed, inhale and lower your feet, and repeat the exercise. This is more difficult than the Alternate Bent-Knee Leg Raise.

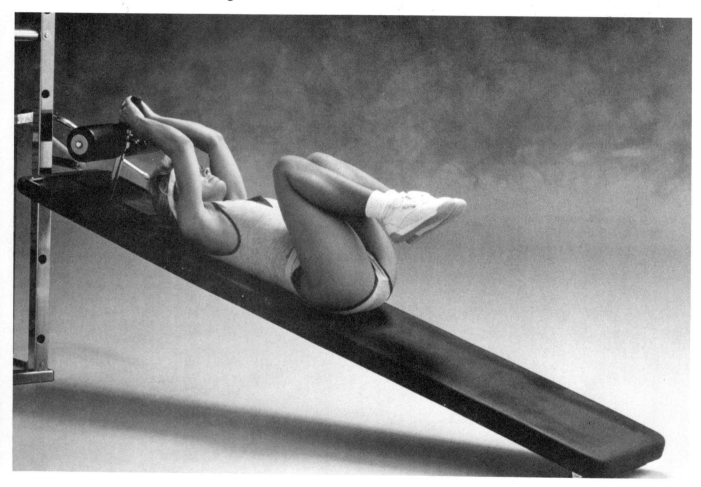

ALTERNATE LEG RAISE

Lying on your back with your head toward the rollers, grasp the handle with both hands, keeping your shoulders flat. Keeping your legs straight, pull one leg up as far as possible over your head. Lower your leg slowly to the starting position and repeat the exercise with your other leg.

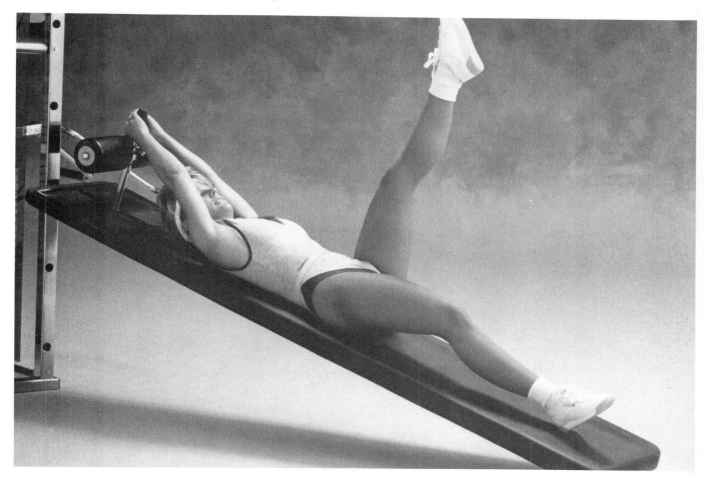

DOUBLE STRAIGHT LEG RAISE

Lying on your back with your head toward the rollers, grasp the handle with both hands, keeping your shoulders flat. Keeping your legs straight, pull both legs up as far as possible over your head. Lower your legs slowly to the starting position.

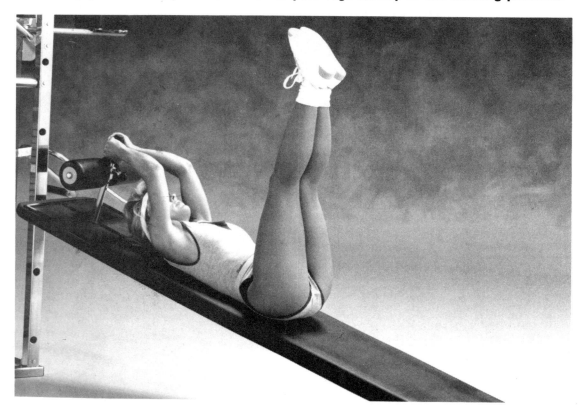

DOUBLE-KNEE LEG RAISE WITH TRUNK TWISTER

This exercise is very demanding—it is not for beginners. Lying on your back with your head toward the rollers, grasp the handle or the rollers. Keep your shoulders flat. Pull your knees up to your chest, twist both knees to one side, point your toes and extend your legs without touching the floor or the board. Rotate through your waist and pull your knees back up to your chest in the center position. Twist and rotate to the opposite side; point your toes and extend your legs—all in one continuous motion. Inhale high in your chest as you draw your knees up; exhale as you extend your legs to the side.

BACK EXTENSION

Lie face down on the board with your head facing away from the machine. Hook your feet under the rollers and place your hands behind your back. Arch your head and back up off the bench until they are parallel with the floor. Inhale. Exhale as you return to the starting position.

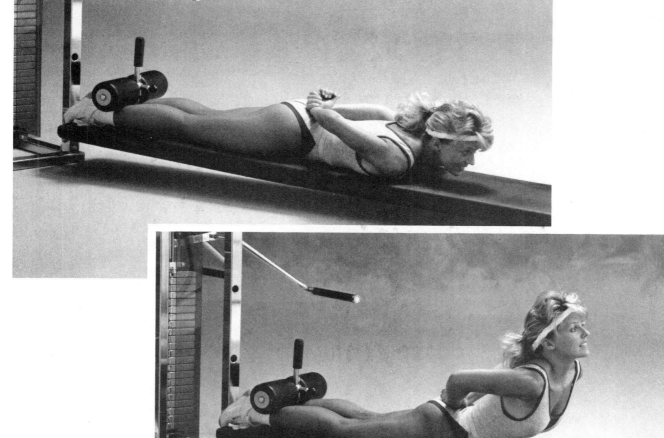

SINGLE BACK LEG RAISE

Muscle groups affected:

lower back muscles, buttocks.

Lie on your stomach with your head toward the rollers. Grasp the handle or the rollers. Keep your hips flat on the board. Raise one leg parallel with the floor while pointing your toes. Repeat with other leg. Maintain control and breathe normally.

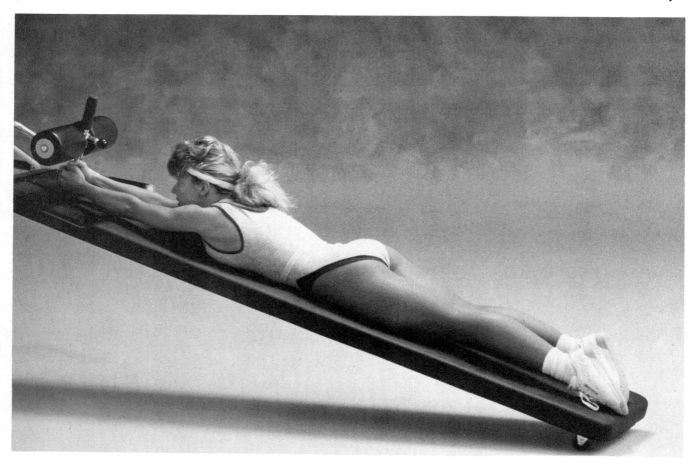

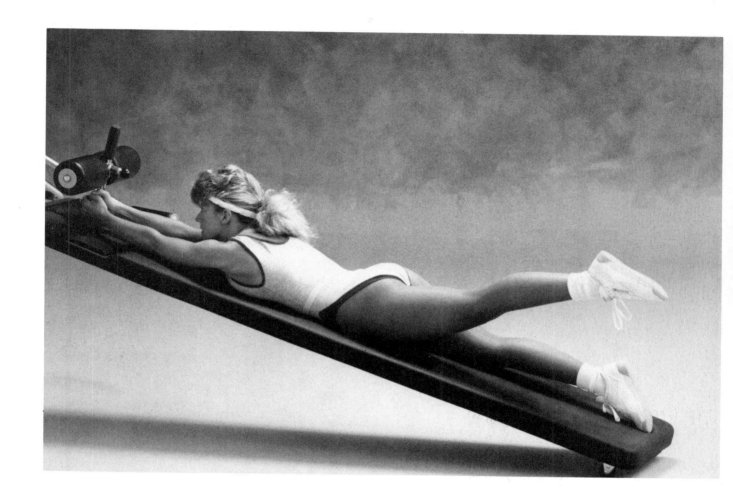

DOUBLE BACK LEG RAISE

Lie on your stomach with your head toward the rollers. Grasp the handle or the rollers. Keep your hips flat on the board. Raise both legs parallel with the floor while pointing your toes. Maintain control and breathe normally.

Muscle groups affected:

lower back muscles, buttocks.

ABDOMINALS AND LOWER BACK

BACK EXTENSION

Muscle groups affected:

lower back muscles, buttock and hamstring stretch (hip).

Facing away from the machine, place your pelvis on the hip pad. Raise your left leg so it's under the roller and place your right foot on the foot plate, pushing slightly to hold your position. Place your hands behind your head with your fingers interlaced. Bend forward and down, exhaling on the way down. Then lift your head and body to a horizontal position, inhaling on the way up. Repeat.

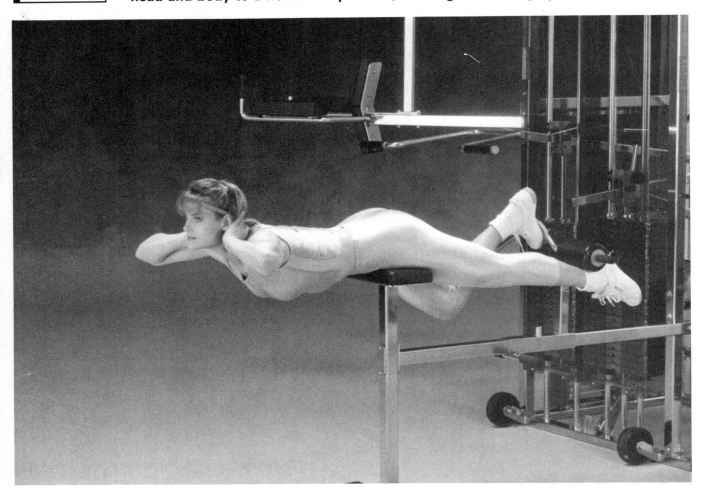

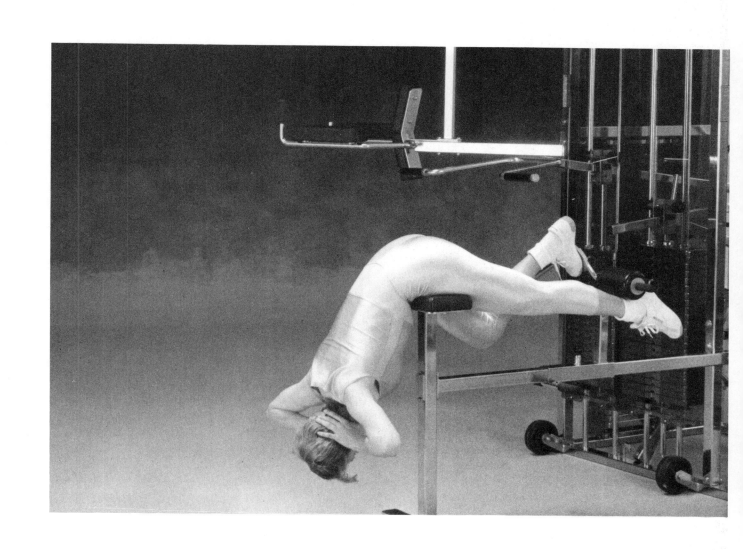

Muscle
groups
affected:

lower back
muscles,
buttocks, and
hamstring
insertion.

DOUBLE BACK LEG RAISE

Facing the machine, place your pelvis on the hip pad. Bend forward and grasp the handle and the foot plate. Raise both legs simultaneously as high as possible. Lower your legs under control and repeat the exercise.

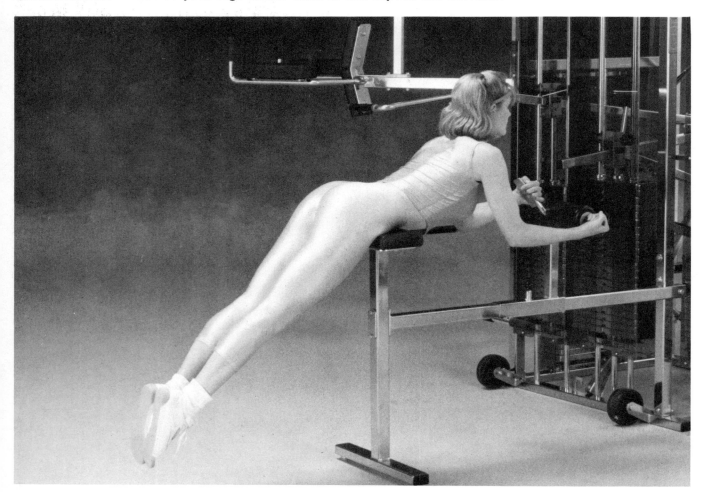

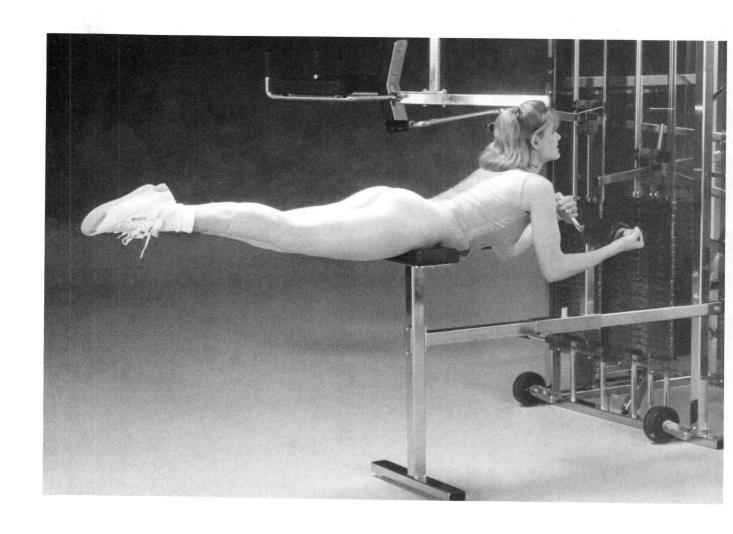

ALTERNATE BACK LEG RAISE

Facing the machine, place your pelvis on the hip pad. Bend forward and grasp the handle and the foot plate. Alternately raise each leg as high as possible. Lower each leg, maintaining control.

ABDOMINALS AND LOWER BACK

ROMAN CHAIR SIT-UP

Sit on the hip pad, facing the machine. Place one foot under the roller and one on top of the roller. Put your hands behind your head and interlace your fingers, or fold your arms across your chest. Bend backward until your back is parallel to the floor. Return to the sit-up position. Inhale going down, exhale coming up. This exercise is for advanced training only. Beginners should not attempt it.

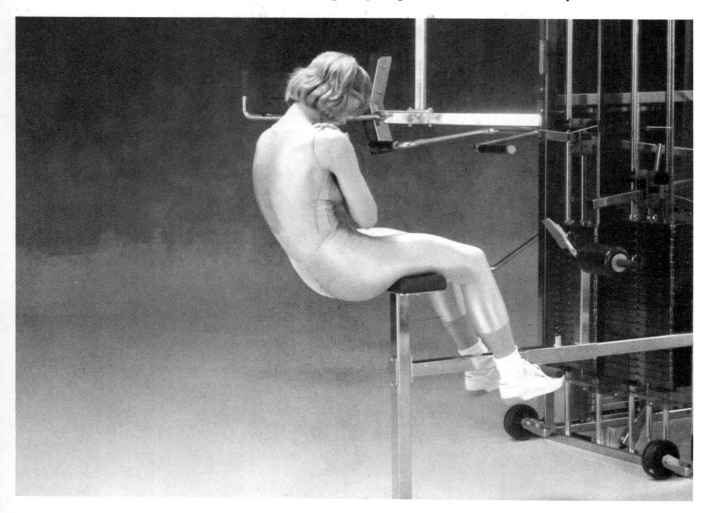

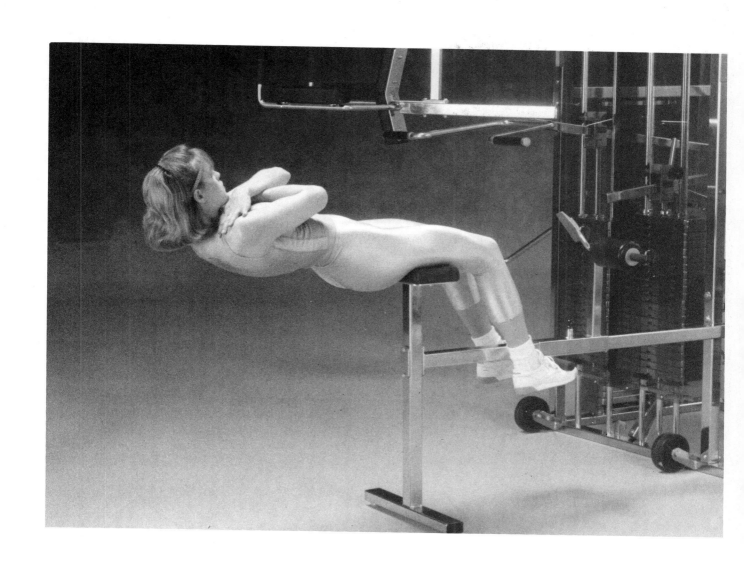

SIDE BEND

Muscle groups affected:

abdominals and external obliques.

Stand with your side to the handle of the chest press. Grip the handle tightly, with your index finger in the bend of the handle. Lift the weight by bending away from the machine, keeping your arm straight. Both feet should remain flat on the floor. Keep your inside leg straight and your head up.

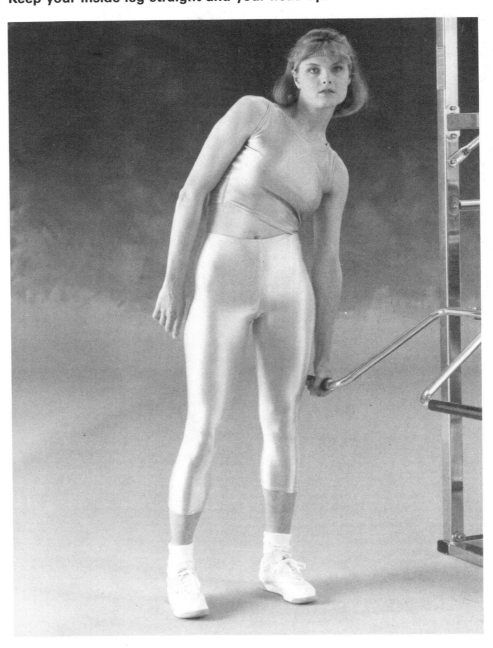

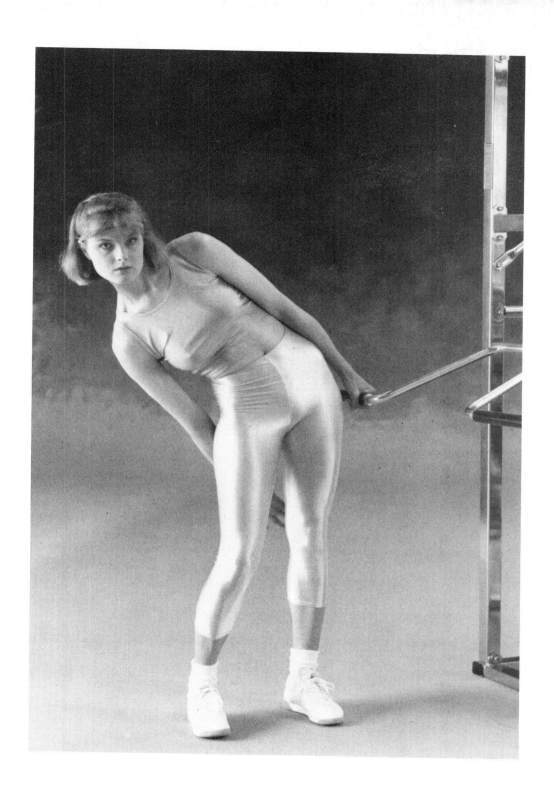

SIT-UP (Using the Bar or Handles)

Muscle group affected:

abdominals.

Sit on the floor facing away from the machine. Grab the bar behind your head, using a shoulder-width grip. Bend your knees. With someone holding your feet, do a curl-type sit-up. Exhale at the completion of the sit-up.

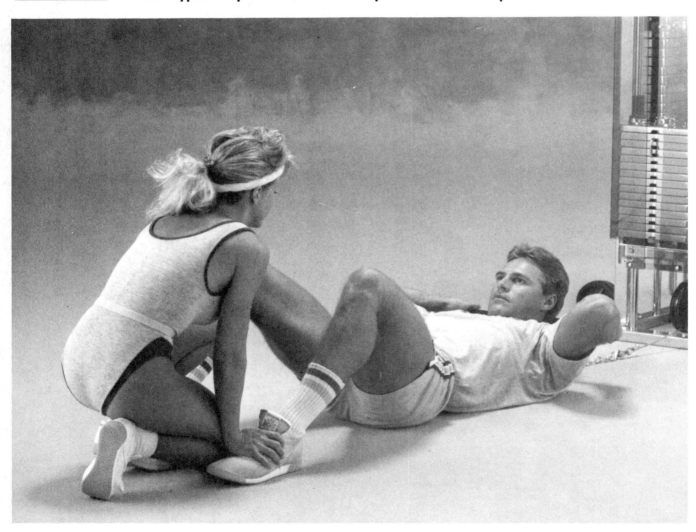

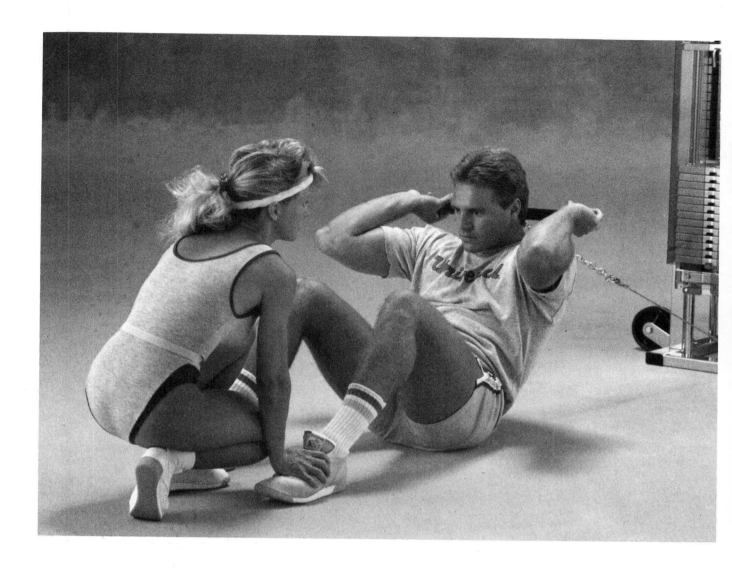

TRUNK TWISTER SIT-UP

Sit on the floor facing away from the machine. Grab the bar behind your head, using a shoulder-width grip. Bend your knees. With someone holding your feet, do a curl-type sit-up, twisting your trunk at the top of each sit-up. Exhale at the completion of the sit-up.

Muscle groups affected:

abdominals, internal and external obliques.

ABDOMINALS AND LOWER BACK

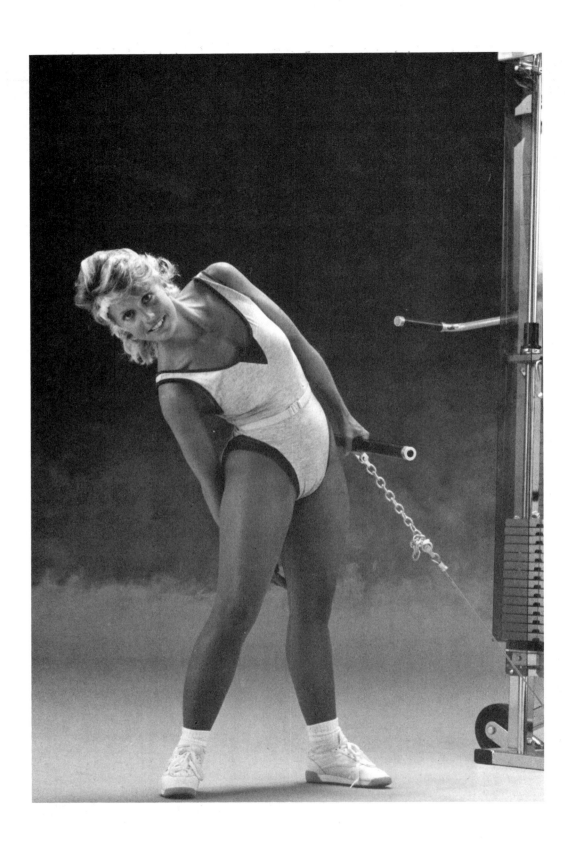

9
HAND STRENGTH

Hand strength is one of the most important, yet most overlooked, aspects of athletic conditioning and performance. In almost all competitive sports, hand strength plays a major role. In football, for example, hand strength is needed for tackling, passing, and receiving. Basketball, too, relies on hand strength and dexterity. In baseball, catching, fielding, and throwing all require excellent hand strength. Golfers and tennis players focus the power of their arms through their hands for power and accuracy. Swimmers need strong hands to pull themselves through the water.

In the past, physical activity was a regular part of our everyday lives and there was no need for special programs for hand strength because people got all the hand exercise they needed milking the cows, chopping wood, and pitching hay. However, times have changed, and most people no longer perform the kind of activities that lead to hand strength. Considering how valuable hand strength can be, it's surprising that more people don't work on hand strength more. The following program will help build up your hands and wrists for all types of sports. This program should be done at least three times per week, and if your muscles recover quickly it can be done daily.

WRIST CURL (Palms Up)

Place your hand on the handle (or both hands on the bar) of the lower pulley station with your palms up. Bend your wrists toward you. Do three sets of fifteen reps.

WRIST CURLS (Palms Down)

Place your hands on the bar with your palms down. Bend your wrists toward you. Do three sets of fifteen reps. (See page 115.)

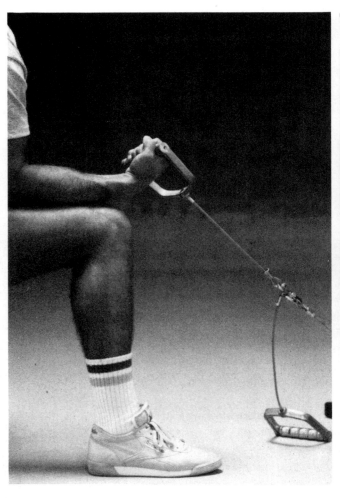
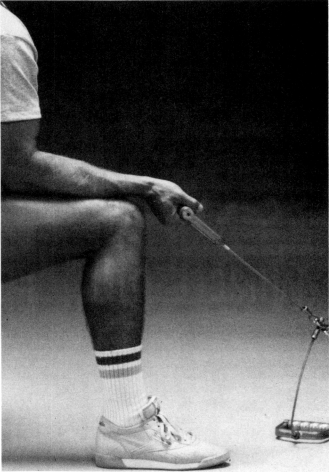

WRIST CURL

Place your hands on the grips with your palms down. Bend your wrists away from you. Do ten reps.

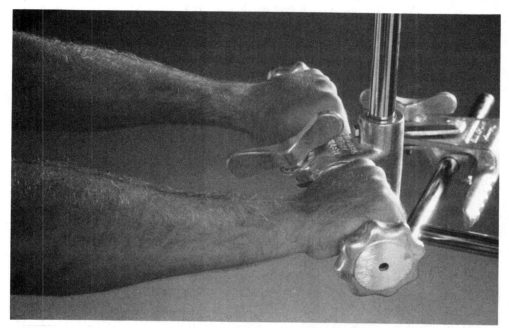

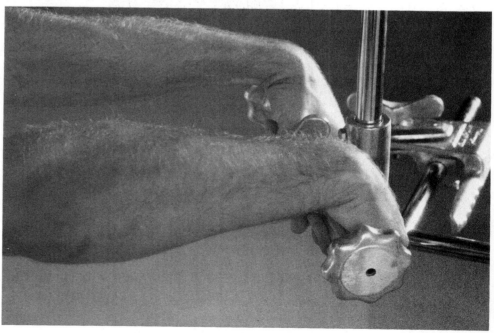

REVERSE WRIST CURL

Place your hands on the grips with your palms down. Bend your wrists toward you. Do ten reps.

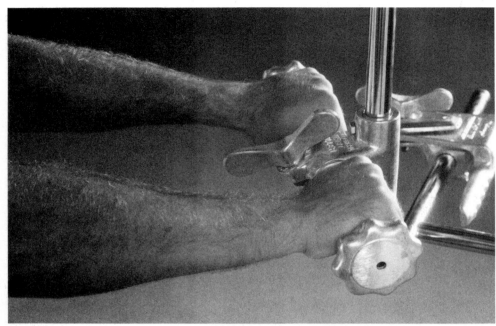

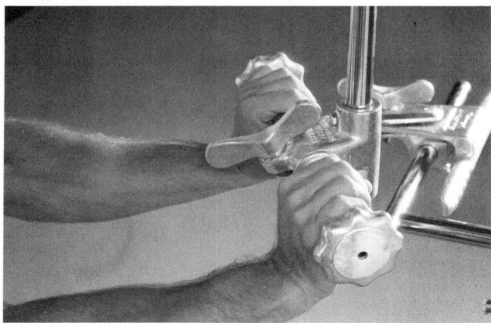

LATERAL WRIST CURL

Place your hands on the doorknoblike ends. Rotate your wrists away from you. Do three sets of ten reps.

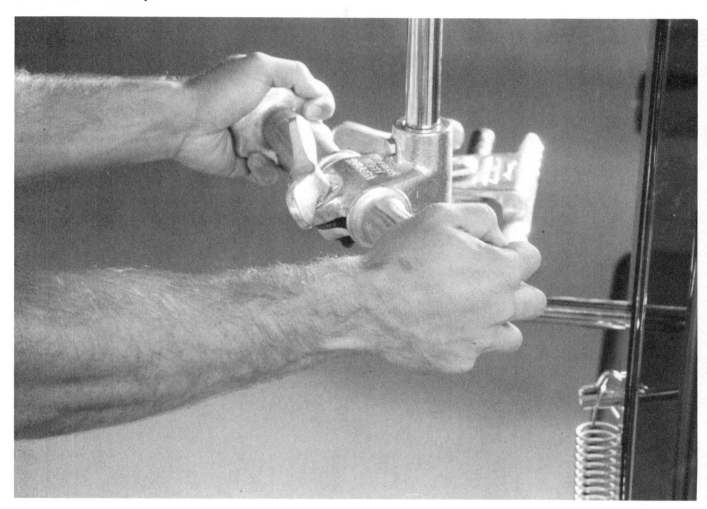

REVERSE LATERAL WRIST CURL

Place your hands on the doorknoblike ends. Rotate your wrists toward you. Do three sets of ten reps.

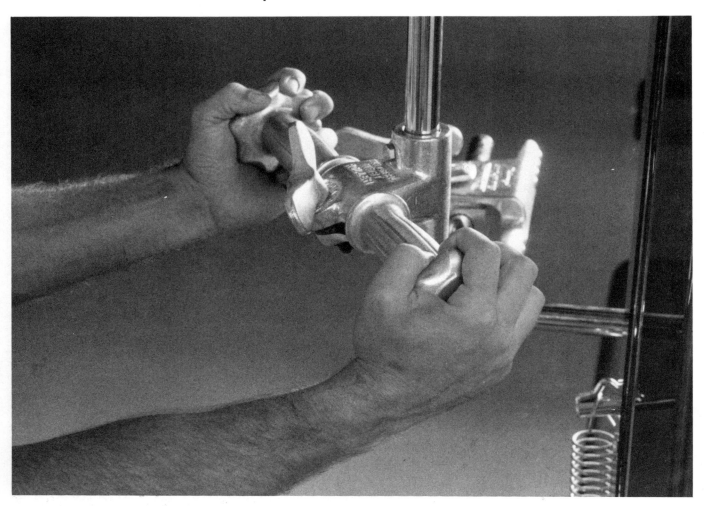

PRONATION EXERCISE

Grasp the handle from the end. Rotate your hand inward.

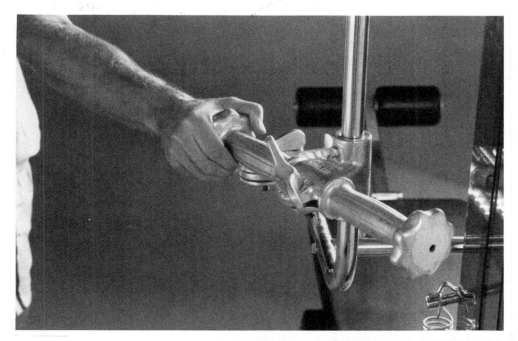

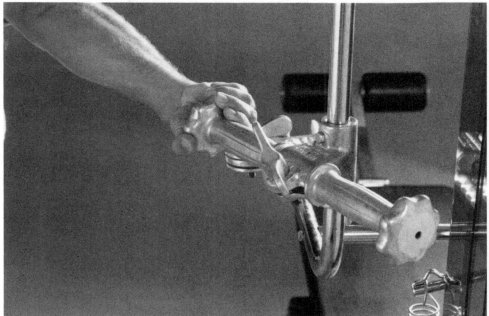

SUPINATION EXERCISE

Grasp the handle from the end. Rotate your hand outward.

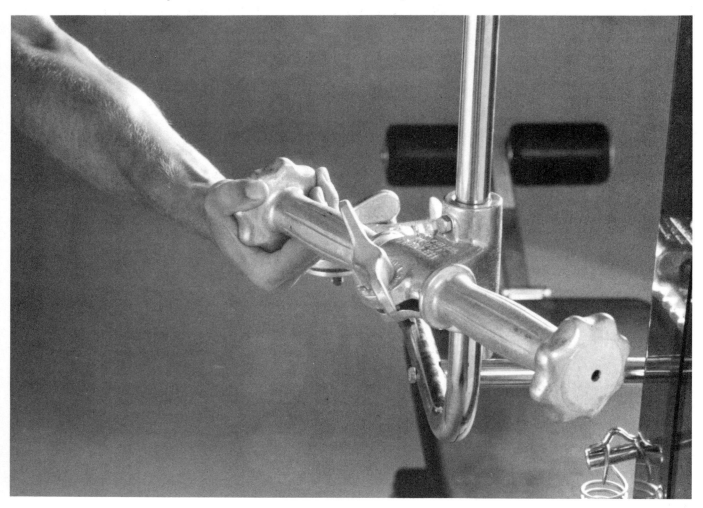

PALMS-UP SQUEEZE

With your palms up, hold the squeezer bars together with one hand and squeeze with the other hand. Repeat using the opposite hand.

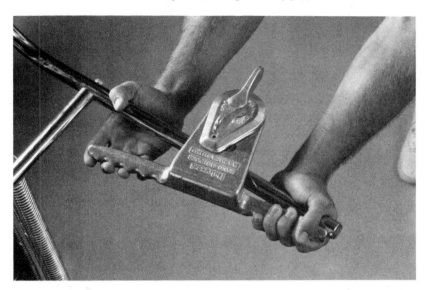

PALMS-DOWN SQUEEZE

With your palms down, hold the squeezer bars together with one hand and squeeze with the other hand. Repeat using the opposite hand.

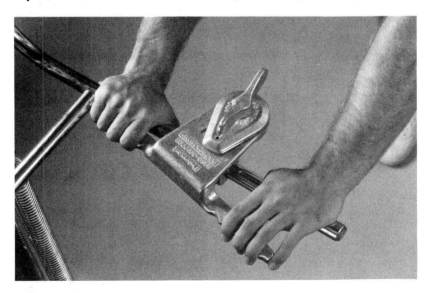

The following exercises enable you to work out your hands when you're away from the gym.

PAPER CRUSHER

Place a double sheet of newspaper flat on a table. Starting at one corner with the heel of your hand in contact with the table, pull the entire sheet into your hand by using your fingers. When you have it in a ball, squeeze it hard ten times. Repeat with the other hand. Doing three double sheets is a good beginning. When you can do the Sunday *New York Times,* your hands are in *great* shape.

BALL SQUEEZING

Get a rubber ball from a toy store, or a tennis ball, and practice squeezing it. Really work at squeezing the ball. This is a good hand-strengthening exercise.

SPRING HAND GRIPPERS

Available at any sporting goods store, this piece of equipment can quickly increase your hand strength, especially if you follow each repetition by doing a wrist rotation.

One-Hand Dead Lift

With a barbell and a considerable amount of weight, this is an excellent exercise.

"Muscle Out" Feats

Use a twelve- or sixteen-pound sledgehammer. Gripping the end of the handle, try to pull the sledge's head toward you using the power of your wrists.

In addition, rope climbing, tug-of-war, and hanging from a horizontal bar will all improve your hands' endurance and strength.

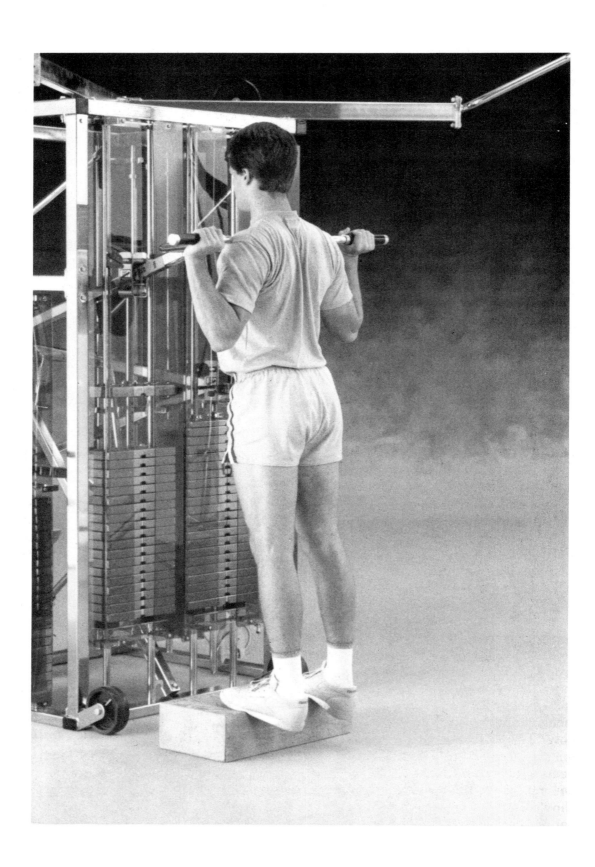

10

WORKOUT ROUTINES AND CIRCUIT TRAINING

In the last few chapters, we have shown how to perform the exercises in Universal's multistation circuit. Now you're ready to begin to set up your training program. The following exercise program should fit your needs whether you are a man or a woman, young or old. The first thing you want to do is weigh yourself and measure the size of your arms, chest, thighs, calves, waist, and hips. These vital statistics provide benchmarks to measure your progress and motivate you to stay committed to your program. ("I've taken two inches off my waist and added two inches to my chest. How can I stop now?") In addition, count your pulse for ten seconds and multiply the number of beats by six to get your resting pulse rate per minute. In the months ahead, you should see a noticeable drop in the number of times your heart has to beat each minute, signaling that your heart is becoming a more efficient machine.

Here are the exercises we'd suggest for an initial fitness program:

1. Chest or Bench Press   p. 68
2. Crunch Sit-Up   p. 140
3. Leg Press   p. 62
4. Front Pull-Down   p. 86
5. Leg Extension   p. 56
6. Hip Flexor   p. 66
7. Forward Shoulder Press   p. 78
8. Double Leg Curl   p. 58
9. Double Arm Curl or Alternate Arm Curl   pp. 98, 99
10. Bent-Over Rowing   p. 94
11. Calf Raise   p. 60

For the first week, you should do twelve to fifteen repetitions of all the exercises using just one weight plate. You may say, "C'mon, I can do a lot more than that." Chances are you can, too. But for the first week, the goal is not to transform yourself into a shining example of athletic perfection. For this first week, the goal is to make sure you have your *form* down pat on the exercises. Improper form will fail to isolate the proper muscle groups, which means that later you may end up working your back muscles when you intend to exercise your stomach muscles. That kind of laissez-faire muscle development program can also lead to injury. So be patient and concentrate on executing each exercise correctly and completely.

After your initial week is complete, it's time to test for your maximum one-time lift capability for each of the exercises listed. Start by lifting the *lowest* weight available at each station. Chances are you'll have no problem. Next, try the next-higher weight, and so on. Increase the weight one or two plates at a time until you reach a weight that you can perform only one complete repetition. Your maximum, then, is the last weight you could lift. You may want to skip the lower weights and advance to a weight nearer what you think your maximum might be. Resist that urge. The method we've outlined here has a built-in fatigue factor that ensures that the weight you use in your program will not cause injury.

PHASE I

For the first six to eight weeks, use 40 percent of your maximum weight to do the exercises in your program. This weight may seem light, but if you haven't worked out recently your muscles need time to adapt to the new stresses you're placing on them. Respect your body enough to give it some extra care in the initial stages of your training regimen. The name of the game here is *progressive* muscle resistance. As your muscles become stronger and you can complete the final reps in your set without difficulty, you can up your weight to the next setting. Remember, it's not where you start, it's where you finish. Also, by starting with a low weight, you're more likely to make advances in your weights, which will keep you motivated to follow your program. Before long, your workouts will become a regular and necessary part of your life. If you bite off more than you can chew at the beginning, you're more apt to become just another fitness dropout. Don't let it happen to you.

PHASE II

Congratulations, you've completed the first six to eight weeks of your program. It's time now to check out your physical data. Record your weight and measurements. Don't be concerned if you've actually put on weight. A weight gain can be deceptive, since muscle weighs more than fat. If your measurements are heading in the right direction, you can feel fairly confident in ignoring the scale.

Record your resting pulse rate and then try the step test described earlier in the book, stepping on and off a twelve-inch bench for three minutes. Record your pulse rate one minute after you complete the step test. The closer this pulse rate is to your normal resting pulse rate, the more fit you are.

It's time again to test your new weight maximum for each exercise. Start by lifting your old maximum. If that's no problem, keep upping the weight one plate at a time until you are unable to complete one repetition. Your new maximum is the last weight you could lift.

Continue with your exercise program using 40 percent of your new maximum as your training weight. Strive always for proper form. After six to eight more weeks of training, you can advance to either the High-Strength Development Program or the High-Endurance Program, which are described in the following sections, or just stay with the exercise in Phase II.

For many people, Phase II will be all the exercise they need. It all depends on your progress and your fitness goals. If you stop making gains, or see a marked decline in your performance, you need to readjust your program. Try incorporating other exercises into your routine that work your muscle groups differently. If you start training for a new sport, you will want to adapt your program to meet the requirements of the new activity. For example, professional football players need to build up their neck muscles much more than most people in order to withstand the bone-jarring impact caused by blocking. If your efforts at firming up and losing weight aren't going as planned, a new workout program might be necessary. But remember, no workout routine can deliver results unless you work out conscientiously.

HIGH-STRENGTH DEVELOPMENT—THE UNIVERSAL ANTAGONISTIC MUSCLE CIRCUIT

If strength is your goal, the exercises in this program are for you. The Universal Antagonistic Muscle Circuit alternately exercises muscle groups that work in direct opposition to each other. For example, an abdominal exercise (sit-up) is followed with a back exercise (back extension) and so on through the entire session. Here's the suggested exercise sequence:

1. Bench or Chest Press   p. 68
2. Front/Back Pull-Downs
   (High-Lat Pulley)   pp. 84–87
3. Double Leg Extension or
   Single Leg Extension   pp. 56–57
4. Double Leg Curl   p. 58
5. Crunch Sit-Up   p. 140
6. Back Extension   p. 149
7. Double Arm Curl or
   Alternate Arm Curl   pp. 98, 99
8. Dipping or Reverse Grip
   Dip   pp. 123, 124
9. Leg Press   p. 50
10. Dead Lift   p. 76
11. Pull-Over or Bent Arm
    Pull-Over   pp. 102, 104
12. Upright Rowing   p. 96

In the basic program, you'll use 70 to 80 percent of your maximum weight and do three sets of five to seven reps. After six to eight weeks, retest your maximum weight and adjust your program accordingly. Feel free to substitute other exercises that work the same muscle groups as those listed. For example, you could occasionally substitute Side Bends (on the Chest Press Station) for Crunch Sit-Ups.

HIGH-ENDURANCE PROGRAM

If muscular endurance is what you're interested in, the following exercise sequence is what you need.

1. Exercise bike or jogging in
   place   p. 182
2. Forward Shoulder Press   p. 78
3. Leg Press   p. 50
4. Bench or Chest Press   p. 68
5. Double Leg Extension or
   Single Leg Extension   pp. 56–57
6. Double Arm Curl or
   Alternate Arm Curl   pp. 98, 99
7. Double Leg Curl   p. 58
8. Front Pull-Down (High-Lat
   Pulley)   p. 84
9. Crunch Sit-Up or Twisting
   Sit-Up   pp. 140–142
10. Upright Rowing (Low
    Pulley)   p. 96
11. Hip Flexor   p. 66
12. Dead Lift   p. 116
13. Back Extension   p. 149
14. Pull-Over   p. 102
15. Back Hip Extension Kick   p. 65

Use 40 to 50 percent of your maximum for each exercise and do three sets of fifteen reps. After six to eight weeks, retest for your maximum for each exercise and adjust your program accordingly. We've described how to perform an abundance of exercises in the earlier chapters. Feel free to substitute other exercises that work the same muscle groups as those listed here. For example, you could substitute Double Back Leg Raises for Back Extensions.

BODY PART DEVELOPMENT, FIRMING, AND TONING

The following program is a maximum workout designed for maximum results. It's definitely not a program for beginners. In fact, because this is such a high-stress program, it has to be done as a split routine. To give your chest a better workout, we recommend you do some **Decline Bench Presses** and **Incline Bench Presses**, which more thoroughly exhaust your chest muscles by bringing new muscle fiber into play. To perform either of these exercises, simply substitute the appropriate bench. The incline bench is slanted so that your upper torso is higher than the rest of your body. Conversely, the decline bench is slanted so that your upper torso is lower than the rest of your body.

MONDAYS AND THURSDAYS

Chest–Shoulders–Arms
Do one set of the first four exercises (1–4) and then repeat the sequence until you have completed four sets. Then do the same thing with 5–8 and 9–12. Use 70 percent of your single-rep maximum and do not rest between sets.

1. Bench Press—4 sets, 7 reps p. 68
2. Bent Arm Pull-Over—4 sets, 7 reps p. 104
3. Decline Bench or Chest Press (use appropriate bench)—4 sets, 7 reps p. 68
4. Incline Sit-Up—4 sets, 21 reps
5. Forward Shoulder Press—4 sets, 7 reps p. 78
6. Lateral Raise—4 sets, 7 reps p. 108
7. Back Shoulder Press—4 sets, 7 reps p. 80
8. Front Pull-Down (narrow grip, palms toward you)—4 sets, 7 reps p. 86
9. Alternate Arm Curl—4 sets, 7 reps p. 99
10. Triceps Extension—4 sets, 7 reps p. 90
11. Wrist Curl—4 sets, 7 reps p. 112
12. French Curl—4 sets, 7 reps p. 82

TUESDAYS AND FRIDAYS

Back
Do one set of the first four exercises (1–4). Repeat the sequence until you have completed four sets. Then do the same thing with 5–8 and 9–12. Use 70 percent of your single-rep maximum.

1. Dead Lift and Shoulder Shrug—4 sets, 7 reps p. 116
2. Back Pull-Down—4 sets, 7 reps p. 84
3. Crunch Sit-Up—4 sets, 7 reps p. 140
4. Back Extension—4sets, 7 reps p. 149
5. Leg Press—4 sets, 7 reps p. 50
6. Double Leg Extension—4 sets, 7 reps p. 56
7. Double Leg Curl—4 sets, 7 reps p. 58
8. Sprinter Kick Back—4 sets, 7 reps p. 54
9. Calf Raise—4 sets, 7 reps pp. 60–61
10. Sit-Up—4 sets, 7 reps p. 160
11. Leg Press (put the heels at the top of the pedals)—4 sets, 7 reps p. 62
12. Back Hip Extension Kick—4 sets, 7 reps p. 65
13. Hip Flexor—4 sets, 15 reps p. 66

WEDNESDAYS AND SATURDAYS

Do at least 30 minutes of aerobic exercises with your heart rate in your target range. For example, you could walk rapidly for three to four miles, swim, or include some distance running at three-quarters speed.

DEVISING YOUR OWN WORKOUT

The programs we've outlined here are the *foundation* for what we hope will become a lifelong fitness program. But if you're training for some specific purpose, you may need a more individualized program. Future books will provide in-depth looks at some specialized fitness programs, but don't overlook the fitness instructors at your gym. Think of them as your partners in health and fitness. They can help you adapt one of our basic programs for your new fitness goals — or create an entirely new program for you.

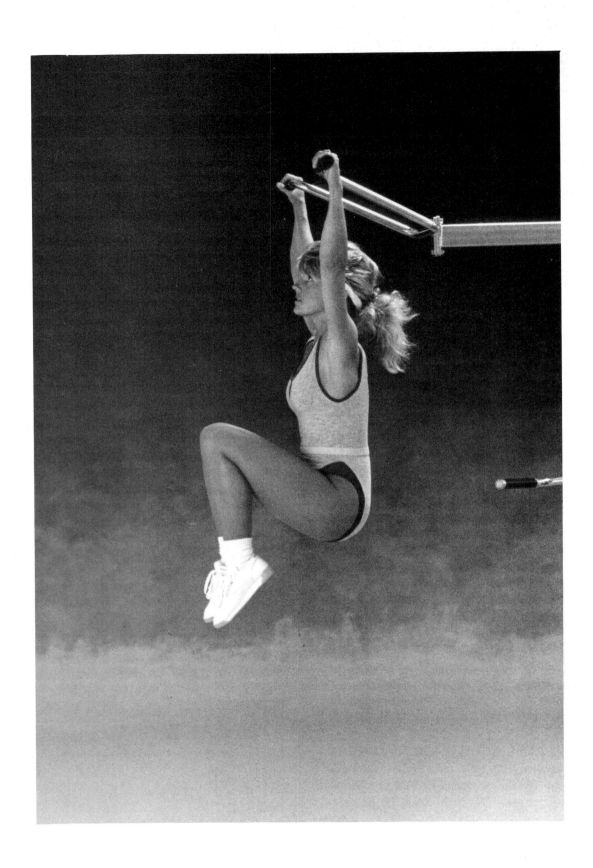

11

AEROBICS AND UNIVERSAL WORKOUTS

It is important to emphasize again that the aim of Universal fitness is more than a strongly toned body. Strong muscles are nice to look at and can help you excel in sports, but that's as far as it goes. What's vitally important is that your heart and lungs are conditioned to supply the energy you need throughout your life. If you neglect this component of the fitness equation, opting for strength gains and body building alone, you may look fit without enjoying any of the benefits of a strong, healthy cardiorespiratory system, including a long, healthy life.

What's needed, in a word, is aerobics. But before we get to the specifics of how aerobic activities complement Universal systems, we should give some credit where credit is due. Dr. Kenneth Cooper has achieved legendary status—and with good reason. His landmark book, *Aerobics,* more than any other, helped spawn the aerobics revolution. We tip our hats to Dr. Cooper for the debt the fitness world owes him. His book, which outlines a point system for aerobic ac-

tivities, is well worth the few dollars it costs.

Dr. Cooper's book details the aerobic value of a host of activities, but for our purposes all you need to know is that you must work your heart for twenty minutes, three times a week, at 60 to 80 percent of its maximum rate to gain aerobic benefit from an exercise. Your maximum heart rate can be determined by subtracting your age from 220. Thus, the maximum heart rate for a thirty-year-old man would be 220 minus 30, or 190. For aerobic training, he would need to keep his heart rate at 114 to 152 beats per minute for at least twenty minutes to gain aerobic benefit from the exercise. Highly conditioned athletes should try to keep their heart rate at the upper end of the range; newcomers to exercise should probably start off at the lower end.

Taking your pulse while you exercise can be tricky, especially if your heart rate is galloping along at more than 150 beats a minute. Here are some additional indicators to determine whether the exercise you do has aerobic benefit. Your aerobic exercise should be intense enough to work up at least a slight sweat on your forehead. If you're jogging, your pace should be brisk enough to noticeably elevate your heart and respiration rates, but not so fast that you can't carry on a conversation with your running partner. If you're gasping for breath, you've crossed the line from aerobic to anaerobic activity. Stop until you've worked off your oxygen debt and then continue at a slower pace.

MODES OF EXERCISE

The activity you choose to develop your cardiorespiratory fitness doesn't matter as much as finding something you will stick with. The ideal activity is something that you enjoy and that fits well into your lifestyle. For example, you probably wouldn't want to begin a swimming program if you do not have relatively easy access to a pool. Nor would you want to start a running program if you were planning to move to Venice, Italy. If you weight train three days a week (Monday, Wednesday, and Friday) do the majority of your aerobic activities on the off days (Tuesday, Thursday, and Saturday). Combining activities in this way is a terrific way to achieve total body fitness.

Let's look at some of the most common—and most effective—exercises you can perform outside the gym.

WALKING, JOGGING, AND RUNNING

Walking is an activity that you can perform well into your later years. Perhaps that's one reason for the tremendous increase in interest in walking. The key for aerobic fitness is to maintain a brisk pace. Strolling along will not give you a strong enough workout. If you have time to stop and smell the roses, you're going too slowly. Brisk walking tones up the leg muscles without placing a lot of stress on the knees and ankles, which is one of the big reasons it has gained so many adherents.

Jogging and running are also extremely good aerobic exercises. If you can cover a mile in eight minutes or less, you're running; more than eight minutes, you're jogging. As you run, your feet hit the ground with at least three times as much force as when you walk. This type of pounding makes your bones and muscles susceptible to stress fractures and shin splints. Therefore, good running shoes are essential. A properly designed running shoe with plenty of cushioning shields your body from much of the impact of jogging.

CYCLING

Cycling works much the same muscles as running, but without the risk of stress fractures. Inclement weather and accidents, however, are always risks when you ride outdoors. You need to cover about four times as much distance cycling as you would running to get the same benefit. Make sure you wear a properly fitted helmet.

For optimal aerobic training, avoid coasting downhill. Instead, switch to a lower gear and maintain a steady cadence. Stationary bicycles provide good aerobic training too. Just make sure that the resistance on the bike is enough to bring your heart rate up to the training range.

ROWING

Rowing conditions both the upper and lower body. Along with swimming, running, and cross-country skiing, it is one of the best all-around aerobic exercises you can do. The key to a good workout is to maintain a steady stroke rhythm.

If you plan to purchase a rowing machine for your home, invest in a high-quality machine that will perform well and hold up under hard exercise conditions. Consider one that is computerized to provide challenge and instant feedback on how your workout is progressing. One computerized rowing machine even has a race mode where you program in an imaginary opponent's racing pace, and has two moving LED bars to monitor your relative racing positions as the race progresses.

SWIMMING

Swimming is an excellent conditioner. Not only does it improve your heart and lungs, it also tones most of the body's major muscle groups. Maintain a steady stroke to keep your heart rate in the training range. To prevent eye irritation from chlorinated or salt water, always wear goggles.

PERIPHERAL HEART ACTION CIRCUIT

As an aerobic conditioner, the Universal Peripheral Heart Action Circuit gives you slightly more benefit in thirty minutes than you'd get running a mile in eight minutes. The difference is that the Peripheral Heart Action Circuit develops all the muscles in your body.

The Peripheral Heart Action Circuit involves alternating upper- and lower-body exercises throughout the entire circuit. This particular sequence of exercises assures that two consecutive exercise stations do not employ the same muscle group as the prime mover. Upper-body muscles are allowed to recover as you exercise the lower body. You use moderate resistance throughout the cir-

cuit. Most people would lift 40 to 50 percent of their maximum one-time lift capacity; trained athletes, 60 to 70 percent. You also use a high number of repetitions (twelve to fifteen) at a relatively fast, intense exercise pace. The key for aerobic benefit is to allow only a short pause (fifteen seconds) between stations. Longer pauses will drop your heart rate out of the training range, canceling the aerobic benefits of this circuit. If your health club is too crowded to allow you to move from station to station in fifteen seconds, you will be better off using the Aerobic Super Circuit (described in the next section) to develop your cardiovascular endurance.

Following is the suggested exercise sequence for the Peripheral Heart Action Circuit.

MULTISTATION MACHINE CIRCUIT

1. Chest or Bench Press   p. 68
2. Sit-Up   p. 160
3. Dip   p. 123
4. Leg Press   p. 50
5. Front Pull-Down (High-Lat Pulley)   p. 86
6. Leg Extension   p. 56
7. Palms-Up Squeeze   p. 171
8. Leg Curl   p. 58
9. Wrist Conditioners (Wrist Curls & Reverse Wrist Curls)   pp. 112–113, 164–166
10. Neck Conditioners (Backward, Forward, Right-Side Left-Side Neck Extensions)   pp. 128–132
11. Arm Curl (Low Pulley)   p. 98
12. Back Extension   p. 149
13. Forward or Back Shoulder Press   pp. 78, 80
14. Hip Flexor   p. 66
15. Reverse or Regular Grip Chin   pp. 118, 120

Aerobic Super Circuit

For many years, the uninformed have constantly made the statement that weight training just can't deliver cardiorespiratory fitness. Wrong! Recent studies by the Institute for Aerobics Research in Dallas, Texas, showed that Universal's Aerobic Super Circuit improved aerobic endurance by 17 percent, increased leg strength by 26 percent, and reduced body fat levels.

In addition, the Aerobic Super Circuit outscored most other aerobic activities. The results were achieved after twelve weeks of training by average, untrained adults in their late thirties. Longer training periods, especially year-round athletic training programs, could show even greater results.

THE PROGRAM

The exercise sequence for the Aerobic Super Circuit is identical to the Peripheral Heart Action Circuit, except that instead of a fifteen-second pause between exercise stations, you engage in thirty seconds of aerobic activity between exercise stations.

After an initial warm-up and stretching period, raise your pulse rate to a target training level with some type of aerobic activity: jogging, running in place, jumping rope, or cycling. Then perform the first weight training exercise as outlined on page 175 for about thirty seconds (normally, twelve to fifteen repetitions). Use moderate resistance throughout the circuit (40 to 50 percent of maximum one-time lift capacity for average persons; 50 to 70 percent for trained athletes).

After the thirty-second exercise you immediately perform one of the aerobic exercises mentioned above for another thirty seconds. Then proceed immediately to the next exercise station without any interval of rest. The entire Aerobic Super Circuit is performed in this manner, alternating thirty seconds of aerobic exercise with thirty seconds of weight training at each station.

The rapid pace of this circuit ensures that each station is quickly vacated, increasing the turnover time so more people can use the circuit at the same time.

The rapid rotation between stations can be accomplished more easily with the use of recorded music and verbal signals. The musical format helps to motivate you and keeps each session moving along smoothly and efficiently.

MORE BENEFITS

This circuit can shape you up in as little as thirty minutes. So if you're pressed for time, you should really consider opting for the Aerobic Super Circuit to fulfill all your fitness requirements. It can save you from having to log miles around the track or streets to keep your cardiorespiratory system in tune.

If you want to be super-fit, the Aerobic Super Circuit can still benefit you. Once you get into condition, you can increase to two to three complete circuits, four times a week, upgrading your weights as necessary.

12

WHAT'S AHEAD IN UNIVERSAL FITNESS

Throughout its history, Universal has regularly updated its equipment and programs to reflect the latest findings in exercise physiology. One such advancement is the universal DVR which enables users to exercise their muscles through a much fuller range of motion than barbells do. But even with DVR, the machines aren't perfect. Each of us has a *unique* force curve—the amount of force exerted at every point in the exercise—due to the differences in the length of our limbs. People with long arms and legs have to move the weight over a greater distance than people with short arms and legs. But today's exercise machines do not provide any means of adapting to these differences. People have had to cope with "one force curve fits all" machines. Soon all that will change.

Universal has launched what may be the most important development in physical fitness in this generation—FITNET. FITNET is a network of electronic resistive exercise machines controlled by a host computer.

One of the advantages of FITNET is that it offers an Individualized Dynamic Variable Resistance mode which varies the resistance in the exercise to fit your unique force curve. Plus, FITNET gives you immediate feedback, enabling you to see how well you are adhering to your exercise prescription and performing your routine. Later, you can receive a printout of your exercise performance results. Best of all, FITNET stores all this data in its memory banks; the host computer automatically generates a data base on its members and updates their records after each performance.

THE FITNET DIFFERENCE

With all weight-lifting equipment, you know how much you're lifting. The amount you lift is known as "load." But as a way of evaluating performance, this measurement falls short because not everyone is the same size and weight or moves the load the same distance.

A better way to evaluate performance is to look not only at the load, but also at how far you pushed it. This is defined as "work." Therefore, if a short person and a tall person both lift the same load, the tall person works harder because he is pushing the load farther.

But even if you consider both load and work, you're still not measuring everything you should because you haven't taken into account how fast the load is lifted. The hallmark of Universal's programs is that all exercises are done using fast, ballistic motions, just as the body performs in athletic competition. The best means to evaluate resistive exercise performance is *power,* which is determined using the following equation:

$$\frac{\text{Load} \times \text{Distance}}{\text{Time}} = \text{Power}$$

If two people lift the same amount over the same distance, both do the same amount of work. But if one did the lift faster, that person would generate more power.

This is why FITNET is so revolutionary. For the first time, people can take into account all important factors that affect exercise performance: load, distance, and time. Figuring these factors into the power equation is the most accurate means of evaluating performance. The beauty of the FITNET system is that all these calculations are done by the host computer — immediately and accurately.

How Fitnet Works

First you are given a fitness evaluation. The results, along with personal statistics — name, address, age, etc. — are entered into the host computer. Next, the instructor chooses from four exercise modes (IDVR, Isokinetic, Fatigue and Pyramid), and a variety of program options to design an individualized exercise program to coincide with your present fitness level, limitations and desired goals.

Then the instructor enters the program into the host computer and gives you a specially coded FITNET ID card.

This card is used to access your program at each exercise station.

To begin your workout session, simply walk up to the FITNET machine of your choice and run your card through the card reader slot located on the machine's control console. This calls up your program from the host computer.

FITNET will greet you and display your program on the LCD readout located on the control console on each machine. As you perform your reps, FITNET gives you immediate feedback about your performance. It displays a range-of-motion indicator, the number of reps performed, and an average power rating or percentage of fatigue. FITNET also provides motivational messages such as "good job" or "keep pushing," to keep you focused on your exercise program.

FITNET also gives you the option of displaying the operating instructions for the proper use of the machine, which can be helpful if you're a beginner or someone who hasn't worked out in a while.

At the completion of your entire workout, you can obtain a printed report by running your ID card through a card reader at the host computer. The report furnishes the following information:

- Average power performed on all reps in a set
- Work performed on each machine
- Best force curve for the exercise performed on each machine
- Estimated calorie expenditure
- Total work performed during the workout session
- Total time spent on the FITNET system
- Comparative data — test, last and best performance
- Normative data — comparing your performance to others

FITNET is certain to become a driving force in the exercise field. No other system provides Individualized Dynamic Variable Resistance training: no other system can supply such accurate information on your exercise performance; no other system can motivate you as well and ensure that you stick with your individualized exercise prescription; no other system can automatically update your program and chart your progress; no other system is FITNET.

THE FUTURE OF FITNET

FITNET is sure to be a hit wherever it is introduced. Because the host computer maintains a data base of members' exercise performance and regularly updates it, health clubs will find it easy to arrange competitions for most calories burned, most work performed, and most improved. For some people such competitions can be terrific motivators and spur them on to greater performance than they might have thought possible.

Because FITNET is computer-based, advances in exercise physiology can be incorporated in the system by revising the software. This kind of adaptability will ensure that FITNET will remain one of the most advanced exercise systems for years to come.

One likely prospect for a new program is one that would adapt the FITNET system for the rehabilitation of muscles injured in accidents or sports. Such muscles often suffer from a limited range of motion. Because FITNET can ensure that you never stress your muscles beyond what is prudent, it would offer an ideal way to systematically build up these muscles to their former strength and range of motion.

APPENDIX: UNIVERSAL WORKOUT RECORD

Name_____ Age____ Height_____ Sex_____

Physician_____ Phone_____

PHYSICAL PROFILE AND ACHIEVEMENT RECORD

Measurements in inches	Starting		1st		2nd		3rd		4th		5th		6th		Ending	
Date																
Neck																
Bust/Chest																
Biceps	L	R	L	R	L	R	L	R	L	R	L	R	L	R	L	R
Forearms	L	R	L	R	L	R	L	R	L	R	L	R	L	R	L	R
Waist																
Hips																
Thighs	L	R	L	R	L	R	L	R	L	R	L	R	L	R	L	R
Calves	L	R	L	R	L	R	L	R	L	R	L	R	L	R	L	R
Weight																
Flexibility (Hamstrings)																
% Body Fat																
Resting Heart Rate																
Blood Pressure																

Monitoring Your Heart Rate

While exercising, it is recommended that you maintain your heart rate within a target training zone to help improve your cardiovascular/cardiorespiratory condition. You must stay within safe limits and not extend yourself over the average maximal heart rates as shown in the Guide. *Be sure to consult your physician before engaging in any vigorous exercise and training, and obtain prior approval of the planned regimen.*

Your approximate Target Heart Rate can also be established with the formula shown below:

(220 − your age) × 60 percent (Conservative Target Heart Rate for the beginner) Example: 220 minus 40 years old = 180 × 60 percent = 108 Target Heart Rate.

(220 − your age) × 70 percent (Intermediate Target Heart Rate)

(220 − your age) × 80 percent (Advanced Target Heart Rate for the well-conditioned person)

It is critically important to begin each exercise period with a warm-up and stretching routine to warm up the heart as well as the muscles.

CAUTION:

Attempting weight training without a thorough physical examination and the physician's approval of the planned exercise regimen could be dangerous and should be avoided.

Do not begin any exercise regimen before having a coach or instructor demonstrate the proper use of the equipment, show the correct lifting and breathing techniques for each exercise, and help you set up a preconditioning program.

Your heart, muscles, tendons, ligaments, and connective tissues should be progressively preconditioned to withstand the possible stress of weight training and help prevent possible injury.

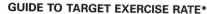

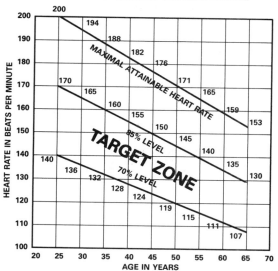

GUIDE TO TARGET EXERCISE RATE*

*According to the principles of exercise programming set forth by the American Heart Association and the President's Council on Physical Fitness and Sports.

WARNING

Serious injuries can occur if struck by falling weights or other moving parts.

You assume a risk of injury using this type equipment. This risk can be reduced by always following these simple rules:

1. Do not use this equipment without *qualified supervision.*
2. Before using, *inspect equipment* for loose, frayed, or worn parts. If in doubt, do not use until parts are replaced. If a fitting fails, you may be struck by falling weights or moving parts.
3. Selector keys must be *fully inserted and locked.* Use only Universal keys—substitutes may cause weights to fall unexpectedly.

4. If weights, pulleys, or other parts become jammed, *do not* attempt to *free by yourself* as weights may fall unexpectedly. Obtain instructor's assistance immediately.

5. To reduce chance of injury, *keep head and limbs clear* of weights and moving parts at all times. Don't be careless, stay alert. Maintain at least a *three-inch clearance* between head and weight stacks in bench work.